Teach Your Child
Yoga

Teach Your Child
Yoga

Fun & Easy Yoga Poses for
Happier, Healthier Kids

Lisa Roberts

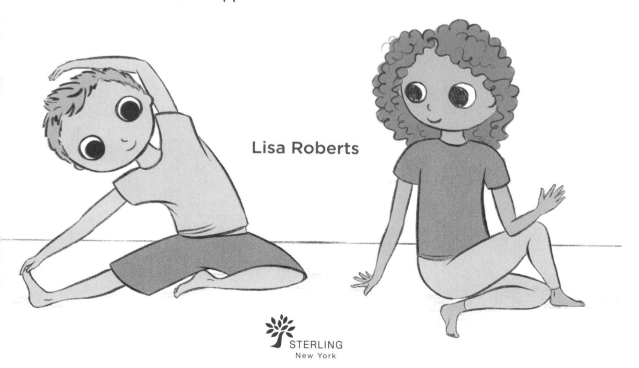

STERLING
New York

STERLING
New York

An Imprint of Sterling Publishing Co., Inc.
1166 Avenue of the Americas
New York, NY 10036

ISBN 978-1-4549-3346-5

Library of Congress Cataloging-in-Publication Data

Names: Roberts, Lisa (Yoga instructor), author.
Title: Teach your child yoga : fun & easy yoga poses for happier, healthier kids / Lisa Roberts.
Description: New York, NY : Sterling Publishing Co., Inc., [2019] | Includes index.
Identifiers: LCCN 2019001928| ISBN 9781454933465 | ISBN 9781454933472 (ebook)
Subjects: LCSH: Hatha yoga for children.
Classification: LCC RJ133.7 .R63 2019 | DDC 613.7/046083--dc23
LC record available at https://lccn.loc.gov/2019001928

Distributed in Canada by Sterling Publishing Co., Inc.
c/o Canadian Manda Group, 664 Annette Street
Toronto, Ontario M6S 2C8, Canada
Distributed in the United Kingdom by GMC Distribution Services
Castle Place, 166 High Street, Lewes, East Sussex BN7 1XU, England
Distributed in Australia by NewSouth Books
University of New South Wales, Sydney, NSW 2052, Australia

For information about custom editions, special sales, and premium and corporate purchases, please contact
Sterling Special Sales at 800-805-5489 or specialsales@sterlingpublishing.com.

Manufactured in Canada

2 4 6 8 10 9 7 5 3 1

sterlingpublishing.com

Cover design by Elizabeth Mihaltse Lindy
Interior design by Shannon Nicole Plunkett
Illustrations by Julia Morris

Teach Your Child Yoga is dedicated to my students, who inspire me to approach yoga with a sense of play and creativity every day.

Contents

Introduction

Yoga has found its way into classrooms, physical education programs, summer camps, and even hospitals. A vehicle for building strength, flexibility, coordination, and balance, yoga practices can be designed to target specific issues, from anxiety to sleep problems, poor posture, and tummy troubles.

Through yoga play, kids explore how amazing the body is and what it can do, boosting confidence, self-image, and self-awareness. Slowing down and experiencing the mind-body connection teaches children a lot about themselves; inner reflection is a wonderful skill to teach our kids, but inner reflection is only valuable when we provide them with tools to support what they discover on their inward journey. Yoga, a practice that explores body, mind, and breath, builds a strong foundation of skills kids can access on and off the yoga mat to navigate stressful situations, promote general wellness, and simply feel happy in body, mind, and spirit.

The bottom line is that yoga is a beneficial tool that kids love. So how can parents share in their child's yoga experience and teach their child yoga? It's simple—*play* yoga *with* your child!

Teach Your Child Yoga is designed so that parents and children can explore yoga together. Regardless of your own yoga experience, this book is a tool to discover and benefit from the magic of yoga with your child. It will grow with your child as his yoga practice, abilities, and developmental needs progress. Whether your child is a toddler or a teen, tips to keep him engaged, safe, and benefitting from yoga are right at your fingertips.

I wish you and your child many fun yoga adventures. Happy stretching!

—Lisa Roberts

CHAPTER ONE

Benefits of Yoga for Children

The word *yoga* comes from the Sanskrit word *yuj* or "connect." What exactly are we connecting? The body, the mind, and the breath—via yoga poses, stretches, meditation, present moment awareness, mindful movement, and mindful breathing techniques.

Benefits of Yoga

These are the known benefits of yoga:

- Increased flexibility, strength, and muscle tone
- Increased mobility, stability, coordination, and balance
- Improved posture
- Improved overall physical fitness
- Improved circulation
- Improved focus and concentration
- Increased mind-body awareness
- Increased confidence, self-esteem, and self-acceptance
- Reduced symptoms of stress, anxiety, and depression
- Improved general sense of well-being
- Improved sleep

Are the Benefits the Same for Children and Adults?

Children who practice yoga enjoy the same benefits as adults (see list on page 2). In addition, yoga supports physical, sensory, cognitive, emotional, and social development in children.

Developing Children and Yoga

Physical Development

Yoga supports rapid growth and body changes, and achieves appropriate physical developmental milestones in children by improving and supporting several areas:

- Fine and gross motor skills, balance, coordination, flexibility, and mobility
- Bilateral integration (see page 215)

- Core tone, stability, and strength
- Posture
- Confidence
- Improved sleep

Sensory Development

Sensory development supports the ability to see, smell, touch, taste, move, and balance. The brain's ability to appropriately interpret input from the sensory systems is called sensory processing. Yoga stimulates the senses and provides input to promote the following:

- Body awareness
- Spatial awareness
- Speech development and oral processing (lip closure and tongue positioning in certain breathing techniques)

- A balance of sensory input to organize and relax the nervous system and modulate arousal levels in children who have delayed, immature, or clinically diagnosed sensory processing disorders

Cognitive Development

The vital skills listed below are utilized in yoga and support children's cognitive development:

- Mind-body connection
- Mental function
- Motor planning (see page 215)
- Language processing and communication skills
- Ability to follow directions
- Ability to focus, learn, and concentrate
- Present-moment awareness and mindfulness skills
- Body awareness and spatial orientation
- Bilateral movement (see page 215)

Emotional and Social Development

Learning how to manage and express emotions—both big and small— is an important skill to help children navigate life's ups and downs. It is equally important for them to learn how to connect with others in a supportive and rewarding way. Here's what yoga can do to help support your child's emotional and social development:

- Develops a self-regulation skill set, or the ability to regulate moods, emotions, reactions, and responses
- Gives your child the ability to shift from reflexive to reflective behavioral patterns
- Provides your child with the ability to self-soothe by learning breathing, meditation, and relaxation skills; reduces feelings of stress and anxiety
- Builds self-awareness, self-esteem, and self-respect
- Teaches your child how to practice compassion and mindfulness with self and others
- Develops communication and leadership skills
- Supports appropriate social interaction
- Encourages teamwork, cooperation, and the ability to participate in a group setting (Chapter Seven, page 214, features fun ways for kids to connect through yoga games.)

Your Child's Learning Style

An important element of teaching is to understand your child's learning style, whether it is visual, auditory, kinesthetic, or tactile. The beautiful thing about yoga is that a well-balanced kids' yoga class incorporates all four styles of learning, allowing your child to benefit and grow in a yoga practice that naturally supports the best style for her. At the same time, she will be exposed to new experiences, ones that she may not ordinarily seek out, and which will encourage development in those areas as well.

If your child struggles in the typical visual/auditory teaching environment, consider creating fun yoga sessions that are themed around what she is learning in school. Learning through movement is particularly supportive of kinesthetic and tactile learners.

The Four Styles of Learning and Teaching Yoga

VISUAL: Visual processors learn through observation. Jump right in and "play" yoga with your child—demonstrate poses and practice together! In addition to demonstration, the illustrations in this book can be helpful when instructing your child in yoga.

AUDITORY: Auditory processors learn through listening. Use verbal directions to support the demonstration of yoga poses. Describe the pose to your child as you practice, and talk to him about the benefits of each pose or practice.

KINESTHETIC: Kinesthetic processors prefer a hands-on approach to learning. Movement, action, and physical activity all support kinesthetic learning, so when your child is moving through a yoga sequence, she will be in learning mode. Support this by theming sessions around school curriculum or other topics your kids are curious about. (For examples, see Shape Yoga for toddlers, page 196, and Bee Yoga for preschoolers, page 199.)

TACTILE: Tactile processors learn through touch and respond well to hands-on activities or projects. For example, using props such as flash cards and creating yoga poses with your child based on topics or skills she is currently learning at school support the tactile learner. And ask for her input! Create and practice sequences together.

Kid Appeal

We've seen that yoga is an essential tool that supports learning and development in children, but how do we get children interested in yoga?

Yoga must be presented in a fun and engaging way so that children *want* to play yoga. Kids' yoga can often be loud and silly, barely resembling an adult yoga class. And that's the point! Kids are not miniature adults, so why should a kids' yoga class be a mini version of an adult yoga class?

Renaming classic yoga postures, from one class to the next, captures your child's imagination, allowing her to experience yoga as a fun journey, while flexing and expanding her mind and imagination as much as her body. Your child can design her own practice or plan super-creative and educational yoga sessions with your guidance, from playful adventures based on beloved characters to lessons about the solar system. No matter what the theme, the underlying goal in kids' yoga is providing skills and tools for children to stretch, grow, and learn in every possible way.

CHAPTER TWO

Teaching Yoga to Children

Think of the guidelines in this chapter as foundational building blocks to create enjoyable and age-appropriate yoga adventures for your child that are safe, beneficial, and *fun*! Here you'll find vital pointers on meeting the developmental abilities and needs of your child and discover how to theme yoga sessions using props, music, journaling, and crafting to create a well-rounded yoga experience.

Familiarize yourself with this instructional chapter and refer to it as needed. However, remember that presence and connection are the heart of yoga, so let go of the concept of *teaching* your child, jump right in, and enjoy yoga adventures *with* your child. If you are in the moment and connecting authentically, you are both practicing yoga, and if you forget an element laid out in this chapter, it's okay.

Kids' Yoga by Age

Just as children's yoga differs greatly from adult yoga, tweaks are necessary to support and engage each of your child's developmental stages. Yoga sessions designed to engage a toddler rarely appeal to a typical tween or teen. Beyond engagement, physical and psychological changes must be taken into account to maintain a practice that is safe, supportive, and beneficial for your child.

PLEASE NOTE: Many important shifts occur at each stage of a child's development. Given that this is a children's yoga book, it will cover only the developmental milestones that apply to yoga.

Children Are Not Miniature Adults

There are a number of major differences between a fully mature adult and a developing child. These are some of the most significant differences between grown-ups and kids to consider when practicing yoga with children:

- At birth, we have approximately 270 bones; a fully developed adult has 206! Developing children's bones are softer than an adult's; some bones eventually fuse together to become one. Never force a child into a yoga pose; allow him to explore his body freely, only offering adjustments if he moves his body in a way that could result in injury. For example, placing pressure on the head or neck.

- Body size and proportions differ greatly between an adult and a developing child; poses an adult can practice easily may not be achievable for a child without the aid of props or support.

- Muscle, bone, and ligament strength differ between children and adults. As bones grow, muscles may become tight until they catch up with that growth. Following a growth spurt, your child's flexibility may change dramatically. Explain that this is normal, and offer modifications to support any changes. Teach patience and demonstrate how your child can use his breath to ease into yoga poses (see page 16 for Teaching Tips).

- Children have thin skin (literally and figuratively), so be mindful of that when using oils, lotions, paints, and so on, as they will be absorbed into a child's skin much more quickly than an adult's. Always be certain that you use nontoxic products that are safe for children. And for figurative thin skin, be mindful of your words, expectations, and tone.

- Children have a higher respiratory rate than adults. As you practice yoga with your child, cue the breath to her rhythm rather than your own. Of course, you can teach your child to slow down her breath, but it may never match yours—think of the difference in lung capacity between yourself and a small child!

- Children have a higher metabolic rate than adults—an hour of yoga right after school is not helpful if your child is hungry!

- Children have immature immune systems. To protect you and your children, keep yoga mats, props, and equipment clean.

- As children develop psychosocial skills, they take learning cues from you! Lead by example to cultivate kindness, patience, love, and respect.

- While children are learning to manage and regulate their emotions, be aware of offering yoga poses or practices that are too challenging or beyond a child's developmental ability. If she becomes frustrated or upset playing yoga, she may not be willing to try again. My motto for teaching all children is observe them, meet them where they are, and build from there.

Yoga and Young Children

Yoga is a sensory experience. The human brain learns everything through the senses, and its most rapid development occurs from birth through age 5. Incorporate music, song, dance, movement, play, and bright, colorful props, such as buttons, bells, balls, and bubbles in your yoga sessions to provide sensory input and support brain development. As your child prepares to meet milestones and learn new things—from identifying colors and shapes, to learning about prehistoric dinosaurs in school—adapt yoga sessions to support his developmental needs.

TODDLER YOGA (18–36 months)

- Toddlers acquire new skills through observation. Verbal instruction is never enough, so it's vital to actually do yoga *with* your toddler! At the same time, you'll be supporting all learning styles—visual, auditory, kinesthetic, and tactile.

- Rapid physical development occurs from birth through age 2. *Never* correct or adjust your toddler's pose, except in the case of potential injury. Allow her to freely explore her body in yoga poses.

- Movement, coordination, and balance can be challenging for young children, as their gross motor skills are developing.

- Fine motor skills are quite undeveloped in toddlers. Use props your child can easily handle, but make sure they are not so small as to be a choking hazard.

TIPS FOR AN ENGAGING TODDLER YOGA PRACTICE

- Songs, music, and lots of movement are great ways to engage toddlers.

- Simple and repetitive poses are best for toddlers! Choose three or four poses and repeat them with simple visual and verbal instructions.

- Use fun and colorful props, such as storybooks (you can theme poses to the story), musical instruments, balls, bubbles, and silk scarves.

- Make noise. If you're a train, say "choo"—or "moo" if you're a cow. Having fun keeps kids engaged!

- Introduce basic breathing. Use a silk scarf, feather, or cotton ball to demonstrate the movement of breath.

- At this age, 15 minutes of yoga is enough for your child. Of course, if he is engaged and having a blast, keep going!

PRESCHOOL YOGA (3–5 years)

- As your 3- to 5-year-old's fine motor skills are developing, introduce crafts, coloring, and simple hand movements into the yoga poses you practice together.

- With a little guidance, the concept of playing and sharing with others will evolve for your preschooler. Yoga games and taking turns leading yoga can help facilitate this growth.

- In the preschool years, gross motor planning and gross motor skills (see page 215) continue to develop.

- For 3- to 5-year-old children, balance can be limited. Introduce simple balancing poses, such as Tree Pose (page 73), using a wall or your own body as support.

TIPS FOR AN ENGAGING PRESCHOOL YOGA PRACTICE

- Imaginative storytelling works well for engaging 3- to 5-year-old children with yoga.

- Teach simple yoga poses and use clear instructions, repeating them as you would for a toddler.

- Use themes that include shapes, colors, letters, and numbers to support learning. (See examples in the Shape Yoga lesson plan on page 196.)

- Emphasize fun and play.

- Introduce and encourage relaxation.

- Allow up to 20 minutes for yoga adventures, 10 minutes for games and songs, and 1 to 2 minutes for relaxation.

SCHOOL-AGE KIDS (5–8 years)

- Between the age of 5 and 8, a child's motor skills and planning improve.

- Verbal processing and the ability to follow instructions and cooperate are greatly expanded at this age.

- 5- to 8-year-olds have great imaginations—tap into this to make yoga fun!

- Bilateral integration (the ability to move both sides of the body simultaneously in a coordinated and controlled manner, see page 215) is developing. Use stickers on the yoga mat or your child's hands to help support this!

- Begin to pay a little more attention to yoga cues (instructions), and help your child get the feel for practicing poses correctly—to the best of his ability, of course!

TIPS FOR AN ENGAGING SCHOOL-AGE YOGA PRACTICE

- Incrementally build on quiet reflection time. If this is too challenging for your child, begin with focus-based activities and games.

- Tap into what your child likes or is learning—popular characters and stories, sports, dinosaurs, superheroes, state capitals, and so on.

- Allow up to 30 minutes for yoga adventures, 10 minutes for games, and up to 5 minutes for meditation or relaxation.

Yoga for Tweens and Teens

When working with tweens and teens, it is important to explain that during practice electronics must be turned off and put away to truly feel and benefit from the yoga experience. It's equally important to get across the concept of connecting to the breath and using it both to move in and out of and to maintain yoga poses. If your tween or teen experiences how powerful the breath is as a tool when approaching a challenging yoga pose, she will (hopefully) take this practice off the mat and use it to face other challenges in daily life.

Tweens and teens tend to be super-sensitive and extremely self-conscious; some may try to force themselves into a pose that is not accessible out of fear of being judged. Communicate with your tween or teen before practicing yoga, and remind him that he has a say in his yoga practice: that he needs to listen to his own body and not force himself.

Teaching Tip

Give your child the confidence to speak up about her yoga practice—it will transfer to other areas in her life! Before teaching yoga to children, I always say, "We are all unique and only *you* are in your body. If something does not feel right, don't do it. Tell me and we will work together to find another expression of the yoga pose that works for you."

TWEEN YOGA (9–12 years)

- Your child is experiencing hormonal changes and fluctuations during this developmental stage.
- Major body changes can result in self-conscious behavior at this age. Be kind, patient, and supportive.
- Give your tween the choice to opt out of poses or offer adjustments to make poses more accessible and/or supported.
- Be mindful that rapid growth spurts effect flexibility, coordination, and balance as your tween adapts to major body changes.

TIPS FOR AN ENGAGING TWEEN YOGA PRACTICE

- Encourage longer pose holds and focus on correct alignment.
- Ask permission before making hands-on adjustments. If you are offering your tween an adjustment or tip, be sure to tell her it is an enhancement and not a correction or indication that she is doing anything wrong.
- Rapid growth equals tight muscles! Use modifications and props to support gentle stretching.
- Introduce challenging and strengthening poses to boost confidence.
- Encourage posture awareness and include poses that lengthen the spine and strengthen the core.
- Explain how yoga practices support the body and mind. Give examples of how yoga (breathing, meditation, poses, and stretches) can be accessed off the mat—for example, at school or before an important game.
- Allow up to 45 minutes for a tween yoga practice, plus at least 15 minutes of deep relaxation and meditation.

TEEN AND YOUNG ADULT YOGA (13–18 years)

- During this period, teens and young adults experience hormonal fluctuations, major bodily changes, and more growth spurts.
- Pressure at school can increase, due to exams, college applications and decisions, sports, part-time work, and so on. A regular yoga practice can help alleviate these stressors.

TIPS FOR AN ENGAGING TEEN YOGA PRACTICE

- Teen yoga is much like an adult practice for *sensitive* adults.
- Nurture teens with patience, kindness, encouragement, and understanding.
- Introduce your teen to different styles of yoga—basic hatha stretches (page 21), energizing vinyasa flow (page 170), or gentle restorative yoga (page 211)—and offer him a choice based on how he is feeling.
- Reserve a large portion of your teen's practice for restorative yoga and deep relaxation.
- Allow up to 45 minutes to practice yoga, followed by 30 minutes of deep relaxation.

Teaching Siblings and Mixed-Age Yoga

Mixed-age yoga can be tricky, but it's not impossible! Older kids may become self-conscious doing the goofy things that appeal to young children, such as meowing in Cat Pose (page 83) or sticking out their tongues for Lion's Breath (page 145). Shift the energy of this self-conscious behavior from worry or fear of being silly to leadership, and empower older siblings by enlisting their help with the little ones. Be sure to include a few challenging options for older kids, too, so they benefit from the practice as well.

Teaching Tips

Enhance your child's yoga experience and keep him safe while practicing yoga with the following teaching tips.

The Breath, the Breath, the Breath

The breath is a superpower that everyone can access. As a yoga practitioner and teacher, I believe it is the single most important aspect of yoga. The breath links the mind to the body; when we breathe consciously, the mind focuses on and controls something occurring within the physical body (breathing). Unfolding naturally, moment to moment (practicing breathing techniques or not!), observing each breath from start to finish connects the mind to the present moment. With practice, some of yoga's philosophic teachings, such as single-pointed focus, meditation, present-moment awareness, and the mind-body connection, can be attained.

Breathing techniques are offered in yoga to help us tune in and center before practicing, and to support focus and meditation skills to maintain a mind-body connection during a yoga class. Here's how to use the breath to support alignment and safe stretching in yoga poses:

- Create space and alignment in the body when preparing to enter a yoga pose. The lungs and rib cage expand to accommodate inhales. Follow nature's lead and use inhales to expand, lengthen, and align the body.

- Maintain alignment and release into a pose using the exhale breath; just like the lungs and rib cage, allow the body to relax and let go on the exhale.

- Breathe fully and mindfully while holding a pose; make incremental adjustments to realign the body on each inhale and relax deeper into the pose on each exhale.

- If it's difficult to breathe in a pose, it's an indicator that the body is being pushed beyond its limits. Back out and find the stage of the pose where breathing is easy and comfortable.

- Linking movement with the breath results in slow, controlled body movement.

- Using the breath as a focus tool can aid balance in tricky balancing poses.

For children 5 and over, I recommend using the "gas in a car" analogy to support linking body movement to the breath: If there's no gas, the car doesn't move, but if there's gas and we hit the gas pedal, it moves! The same goes for yoga: The body only moves with an in breath or an out breath. Encourage your child to relax even when his muscles are active, maintaining engagement, as instructed, yet softening his body with each exhale. The ultimate goal is to create strong poses in yoga that are natural and not forced. Using the breath as a tool can help to achieve this.

Children under the age of 5 (and as old as 8) may have trouble making the mind-body connection, and that's okay; it will fall into place when they are ready. Teach young children to connect to the breath by playing with feathers and bubbles, and cue slow, turtle-like movements for yoga poses. Once the mind-body connection clicks in, they'll be well prepared and ready to breathe and move skillfully.

I tell my students that super-challenging yoga poses—the ones they think they'll never be able to do—*are* attainable when they're approached from a state of relaxation and complete control. Flexibility plays a role in achieving the full expression of many yoga poses, but the ability to be focused, relaxed, and in complete control of the breath is still the most important element. The breath really is a superpower!

Equipment and Props

You don't need fancy equipment to practice yoga. If your child loves yoga and you don't mind investing in her passion, a yoga mat, two yoga blocks, a yoga strap, and child-sized bolster are great tools to purchase. Remember, your child is growing, and good-quality mats last a long time. Skip the cute kid-sized yoga mats and invest in a standard-sized one, unless space is an issue. Carpet squares are a great alternative to a yoga mat in small spaces.

To engage the senses, props should be eye-catching, colorful, and fun. Here's a list my favorite props for kids' yoga:

- Musical instruments—shaker eggs, maracas, bells

- Masks (purchase or craft and theme your session around your masks)
- Puppets—hand or finger puppets (also great for theming)
- Face paint (be sure to use nontoxic, washable paints)
- Plastic toys (select a toy and create a pose)
- Small beanbags
- Hula hoops
- Stickers
- Foam shapes
- Silk scarves
- Streamers
- Picture and story books
- Flash cards or colorful images on card stock

Keeping Your Child Safe

- Clean props and mats after each use. (Use a cloth dipped in warm water and mild detergent or use disinfecting wipes.)
- Make sure that props are the right size for your child.
- Be aware of accessories such as bulky beads, a headband, or sunglasses that may need to be removed before practicing yoga.
- If shoes must be worn, be sure that your child's shoelaces are tied before practicing yoga.

Connecting and Communicating with Your Child

- Engage your child in her yoga sessions. What does she like? What does she want to do? What did she enjoy last time? Acknowledge what she enjoys by offering it within the practice, and introduce new ideas and techniques to build on those skills.
- Praise and encourage effort, attentiveness, involvement, and cooperation.
- Focus on what your child *can* do rather than what she cannot. Praise and reward effort over outcome.
- Empower your child by offering choices and involvement in her yoga practice.

- Explain how the different poses and activities benefit your child's body and mind.
- Use positive and empowering language.
- Encourage your child to support and praise her siblings and peers.

Themes

When it comes to kids' yoga, there are plenty of universal themes that are limited only by your—and your child's—imagination. Dig deep. You may be surprised by all the fun ideas you come up with!

POPULAR KIDS' YOGA THEMES

- Music
- Festivals and world events (solstices, Olympics, World Cup, etc.)
- Holidays (Valentine's Day, Halloween, etc.)
- Seasons
- Beach
- Park
- Jungle and rain-forest adventures
- Farm animals

THINKING OUTSIDE OF THE BOX

- Educational themes: state capitals, dinosaurs, math (counting, number/value recognition, solving math problems), spelling (letter recognition, learning sight words, yoga spelling-bee competitions), solar system, botany, world cultures, world animals, world history, local history
- Popular children's superheroes, TV, movie, and storybook characters

Music

Music and songs are engaging and foster learning, breathing, and a positive connection with fellow yogis.

- Sing popular songs and create yoga poses to go with the song.
- Research nursery rhymes from another era or culture and open young minds to history and different ways of life.

- Change the words of popular nursery rhymes. Here are two that always get a smile from the kids I teach: "Row, row, row your boat gently down the stream. If you see an alligator, don't forget to scream—AAHHHH!" or "Jack and Jill went up the hill to practice outdoor yoga. Jack reached for the sun. Jill touched toes to bum. And they felt amazing and wise as Yoda."

Arts and Crafts

From mask making to coloring mandalas, arts and crafts allow children to express creativity. Incorporating a child's creation in his yoga class, such as a paper boat for Belly Breathing (page 140), gives him a sense of ownership of his yoga experience. Here are some more fun arts and crafts ideas for kids' yoga:

- Make puppets, paper boats, hats, or masks.
- Use pipe cleaners to re-create favorite yoga poses; glue on eyes to make yoga characters that kids can keep.
- Color or design and color your own mandalas.
- Make eye pillows; socks and rice work well for this activity.
- Draw or journal about yoga experiences and adventures after class.

Journaling

Journaling encourages inner reflection and develops self-awareness. It may be used as a tool to encourage your child to explore how he feels after his yoga practice, and to help create awareness of "off the mat" uses for yoga. Journaling is not limited to writing—your child may prefer to draw or tell a story about his yoga experience.

Games

Yoga games support social, cognitive, and physical development, and are a fun way to review yoga poses at the end of a yoga session. Chapter Seven (page 214) features twenty-five fun yoga games for you and your kids.

CHAPTER THREE

Basic Posture Guide

The basic posture guide features fifty poses, including tips and modifications to make them accessible to kids of all ages. The poses are arranged by the position that gives the best access to the pose—whether it is seated, standing, prone (on the belly) or supine (on the back)—and is further defined by the category it falls under to help you better understand the benefits for you and your child. These are the eight categories of yoga poses and their benefits:

1. HIP STRETCHES support healthy mobility in the hip joints and stretch, support, and strengthen the lower back.

2. CHEST OPENERS expand and stretch the chest, open the shoulders to correct hunching, and create more space in the chest to support deeper and fuller breathing.

3. CORE STABILIZERS strengthen, tone, and stabilize the core.

4. TWISTS tone core muscles and support rotation, mobility, and flexibility of the spine. Twists gently stimulate the internal organs to support healthy digestion.

5. BALANCING POSES target core stability, balance, coordination, and develop mental focus.

6. BACKBENDS stretch the front side of the body (thighs, groin, belly, chest, and shoulders) and flex, lengthen, and strengthen the spine. Backbends are energizing and direct your attention outside of yourself.

7. **FORWARD BENDS** counter backbends, stretching the back side of the body and the legs (calves, hamstrings, hips, lower back, mid-back, upper back, and shoulders). Forward bends compress the front side of the body to gently massage the internal organs, and quiet and calm the mind by directing awareness away from the outside world toward inner reflection.

8. **INVERSIONS** strengthen upper back muscles, tone and stabilize the core, and develop balance skills. Requiring intense focus, inversions quiet chatty minds. They also serve as a subtle reminder to view things from a different perspective.

Each pose is illustrated and accompanied by kid-friendly instructions to read to your child as she practices. Adjust the level of instruction and adapt the poses according to your child's age and ability (see page 7 for developmentally appropriate yoga tips). Detailed cues help older kids and parents to safely align in a pose, but they will not work for young children, who are more responsive to visual cues: Make a shape with your body and encourage your child to do the same, offering minimal and simple verbal instruction.

As your child matures, your approach can be a little more detail oriented in terms of instruction and alignment. Introduce cueing the link between body movement and the breath for school-aged children as a tool to move safely while transitioning in and out of poses, as well as while holding a pose. Strongly encourage alignment awareness and the use of modifications, as needed, for tweens and teens. The two single most important analogies I offer students—from ages 6 to 96—are very relatable to children:

LEGO®: Yoga is just like Lego: Build one block at a time until you create your masterpiece.

GOLDILOCKS AND THE THREE BEARS: Practice the poses in stages, building from the ground up. As you move through each stage, notice how you feel—

testing just as Goldilocks did: Maybe the early stage of the pose is cool and the fullest expression is hot. Although your child may be able to move his body into the fullest expression of a pose, it may not feel good, or he may not be able to sustain the pose without creating stress or tension. Encourage him to reflect on this and find the stage and expression of the pose that feels just right to him.

Hold poses for three to five rounds of breath, or flow in and out of poses in vinyasa style (linking movement to breath). Breathing with awareness supports the mind-body connection, helps your child to safely move deeper into a pose when her body is ready for it, and indicates whether or not she is pushing too far. If you or your child cannot breathe properly in a yoga pose, you need to back out. Think Goldilocks! Which stage of the pose felt just right? And remember, if you practice a pose on one side, balance the body and practice on the other side, too!

Five additional names are provided for each pose under "Reimagine the Pose!" but there is absolutely nothing wrong with using the original names! Camel can be Camel, and Happy Baby certainly looks like a happy baby. Additional names for the poses are simply suggestions—ways to inspire a fun and creative yoga session with your child. Feel free to come up with your own names for the poses. The more inventive and playful your yoga sessions are, the more your child will want to engage in the practice. Remember, yoga is not only about stretching the body—it's about stretching the mind and imagination, too!

If a prop is required to safely practice or modify a pose, it will be listed. If you don't have access to yoga props, no worries, the following suggestions are handy substitutions:

- YOGA BLOCK: Books, folded towels or blankets, or a small, firm cushion
- YOGA BOLSTER: Pillow, folded towels or blankets (stack as many of these as needed)
- YOGA STRAP: Belt, sport band

There are many yoga poses and variations that are not featured in this book. However, it is a great starting point to introduce your child to yoga and provide him with a beneficial and well-rounded yoga experience. You can design your own practice by selecting poses from the pose guide, or, if you prefer a fun themed sequence or one that has been designed to support a particular goal, look for "See this pose in a lesson" to be directed to kid-friendly sequences designed for each age range or to target the following:

- Focus
- Stress busting
- Energy equalizing
- Chilling out

- Good posture and strong cores
- Allergies and colds
- Digestive support
- Positive body image

SEATED POSTURES

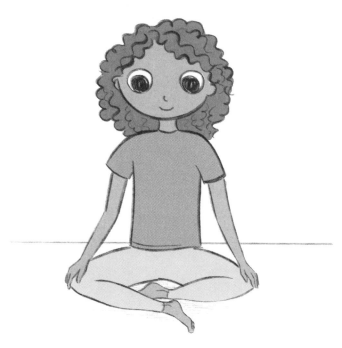

Easy Pose
(following page)

EASY POSE

Sukhasana

What Is Easy Pose and How Does It Help?

Easy Pose is a simple cross-legged pose that gently stretches the hips. It is an ideal pose for practicing breathing techniques, meditation, and upper body stretches. Face, neck, shoulder, arm, wrist, and spine stretches can all be practiced in Easy Pose.

 Simple Steps for Kids

* see page 25 for pose illustration

- Sit on your yoga mat.

- Bend your knees, crossing one ankle in front of the other.

- Allow your knees to open toward the floor.

- Rest your hands on your thighs or knees.

- Press your butt downward, into the floor, and feel your spine lengthen as the crown (top of your head) reaches for the ceiling.

TIP: Kids typically gravitate toward placing the dominant foot in front. To balance this gentle hip stretch and benefit both hips, cue your child to switch the front foot each time he sits in Easy Pose. Encourage him to do this even when not practicing yoga to help break habits that may lead to postural imbalance over time.

》 See this pose in a lesson: stress busting (page 167), energy equalizing (page 170), chilling out (page 173), good posture and strong core (page 177), digestive support (page 188), beach adventure (page 202), partner (page 206), teen restorative (page 211)

Reimagine the Pose!

Queen-Bee • Noodles in a Pot • Crisscross Yoga Sauce • Elevator • Meditation Master

BOUND ANGLE

Baddha Konasana

What Is Bound Angle and How Does It Help?

Bound Angle Pose gently stretches the hips, groin, and inner thighs.

 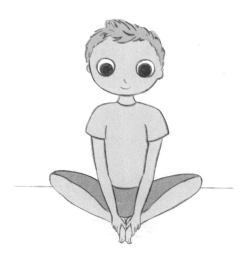

Simple Steps for Kids

- Sit on your yoga mat.

- Bring the soles of your feet together so that they touch, with knees open out toward the floor.

- Wrap your hands around your feet, using your thumbs to grip the inner arches; palms and fingers rest on the top of each foot.

- Straighten your arms and gently pull upward and away from your feet. Notice your spine lengthen.

- Find a sweet stretch that feels *just right*! Draw your heels close to your body to intensify the stretch, and then move them away from your body to ease the stretch.

Modifications

This pose can be uncomfortable for rapidly developing bodies. To ease the intensity of the stretch, place yoga blocks beneath the knees to support them.

Variations

FLYING BUTTERFLY

- Take flight! Gently rock your knees up and down.

STRETCHING BUTTERFLY
(additional core-stabilizing benefits and leg stretches)

- Grip the big toe with the index and middle fingers, or grip the outer edge of each foot with your hands; lift and extend one leg at a time to stretch your butterfly wings.

- For a *big* core and balance challenge, stretch both wings at the same time!

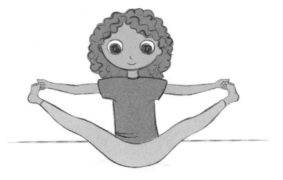

stretching butterfly

SNOOZING BUTTERFLY
(additional forward-bend benefits)

- *Inhale:* Gently pull on your feet to lengthen your spine. *Exhale:* Fold the upper body forward and over your legs. Hold and breathe, relaxing the body a little more with each exhale.

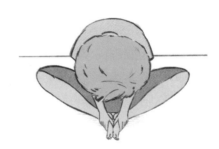

snoozing butterfly

RECLINED BOUND ANGLE

- From a reclined position, bend your knees and place your feet on the floor with the inner knees and feet touching. *Inhale.*

- *Exhale:* Gently open your knees out and down toward the floor. Soles of the feet touch as the knees continue to fall open. *Relax.*

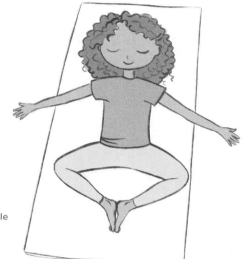

reclined bound angle

» **See this pose in a lesson:** chilling out (page 173), allergies and colds (page 184), digestive support (page 188), shape (page 196), bee (page 199), teen restorative (page 211)

Reimagine the Pose!

Butterfly ▪ Bat ▪ Stingray ▪ Bird or Flying Dinosaur ▪ Baseball Diamond

STAFF POSE
Dandasana

What Is Staff Pose and How Does It Help?

Staff Pose looks simple enough, but it is actually a strong pose that engages the whole body and supports core stability and posture alignment.

 Simple Steps for Kids

- Sit on your yoga mat with your legs extended straight out in front of you.
- Place your hands, palms down and fingers forward, on the floor beside your hips.
- Gently press your hands and butt into the floor, as if you were trying to push the floor away.
- Relax your shoulders away from your ears, as your spine lengthens and your crown reaches to the ceiling.
- To engage the muscles in your feet and legs, flex your feet and pull your toes toward you.

Modifications

Be mindful that tweens and teens experience rapid growth spurts! Cue a gentle bend in the knees or place a supportive prop, such as a rolled-up towel or yoga mat, under the knees to help support tight hamstrings.

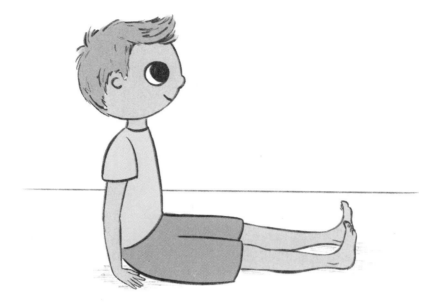

»» See this pose in a lesson: focus (page 163), good posture and strong core (page 177), partner (page 206), teen restorative (page 211)

Reimagine the Pose!

Letter L · *Waterfall* · *Sorcerer's Staff* · *Magic Wand* · *Open Sandwich*

SEATED FORWARD FOLD

Paschimottanasana

What Is Seated Forward Fold and How Does It Help?

Seated Forward Fold is Staff Pose (page 30) with the added benefit of a forward bend—directing the attention inward to calm and quiet busy minds, while gently stretching and releasing the legs and back side of the body.

 Simple Steps for Kids

- Begin in Staff Pose.

- Reach arms up, framing your face.

- *Inhale:* Lengthen your torso and arms from hips to fingertips.

- *Exhale:* Gently fold from the hips and reach your hands toward your feet.

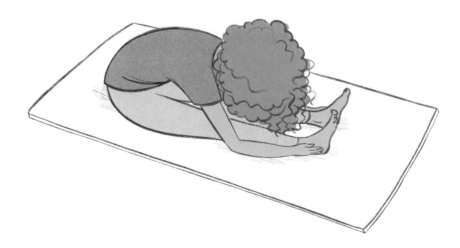

TIP: It is important to maintain a long spine in this forward fold. It doesn't matter if your child's hands don't reach her feet—reaching the knees, shins, or ankles each is acceptable, as long as she continues to lengthen her spine. With practice, patience, and using the breath as a tool, she may eventually reach her feet.

Modifications

Tight tweens and teens may need extra help with Seated Forward Fold.

- **USE A STRAP:** Loop a strap around the feet and gently pull on the strap to guide the torso toward the legs.

- **SUPPORTED SEATED FORWARD FOLD:** Rest a prop such as a bolster or exercise ball on top of the extended legs and relax the upper body over this support.

›› See this pose in a lesson: energy equalizing (page 170), bee (page 199), beach adventure (page 202), partner (page 206), teen restorative (page 211)

Reimagine the Pose!

Sandwich • Treasure Chest • Woodchopper • Apply Sunscreen (Don't forget your toes!)

Horseback Rider (strap modification for reigns)

BOAT

Navasana

What Is Boat and How Does It Help?

Boat is a seated balancing pose that helps to build strong core muscles to support the body.

 Simple Steps for Kids

- Begin in Staff Pose (page 30).

- Place your feet on the floor in front of your hips, knees pointed straight up like tents.

- Grip the back side of your thighs with your hands and gently pull back, to lengthen your spine and expand your chest.

- Lift both feet off the floor and flex them; your knees remain bent for this stage.

- Gently pull on your thighs to realign your spine and feel the muscles in your belly begin to fire up—this is your core working to maintain the pose.

- Try straightening your legs, one at a time, and then both if you can.

- Release the grip on your thighs and reach your hands and arms forward (relax your shoulders away from your ears).

- If this feels good and your core is still working to hold this shape (see Tip on page 35), reach your arms up by your ears—making a V shape with your body.

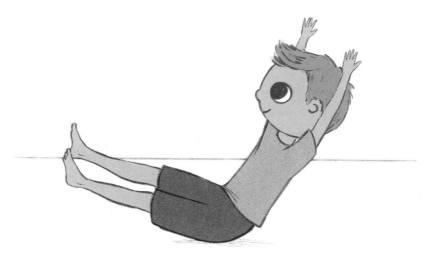

TIP: Watch your child's back! Be sure his core remains engaged while holding this posture. If you notice his lower back sagging or collapsing, he has most likely stopped engaging his core. Direct him to the stage in this pose where he maintained core control and breathing was comfortable. Work incrementally toward the final stage of the posture. Remember, he is getting a strong core workout and balance challenge at each stage!

» **See this pose in a lesson:** focus (page 163), positive body image (page 191), partner (page 206)

Reimagine the Pose!

Letter V ▪ *Bowl* ▪ *Canoe (or any kind of boat)* ▪ *Rower* ▪ *Nest*

HEAD TO KNEE POSE

Janu Sirsasana

What Is Head to Knee Pose and How Does It Help?

Head to Knee Pose reaps the benefits of a forward bend and hip stretch in one simple pose. The legs are also stretched in this pose, and by practicing it on each side, kids learn that the left and right side of their body can feel quite different. Lucky we have yoga to help balance that out!

Simple Steps for Kids

- Sit on a yoga mat with the right leg straight but angled slightly away from your body.

- Bend the left knee and place the sole of your left foot along the inseam of your right thigh.

- Turn your torso to the right, aligning it with the extended leg.

- *Inhale:* Lengthen the spine and reach your arms up to frame your face.

- *Exhale:* Hinge from your hips and lengthen your torso over the extended leg. Hands reach toward the foot.

- Repeat on the left side.

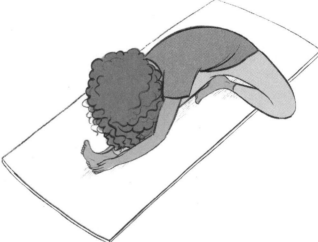

TIP: This is called Head to Knee Pose, and with practice and patience, your child may eventually touch her head to her knees. If she doesn't make this connection, it's not a big deal. The same goes for the hands and feet—it's okay if her hands reach the knees, shins, or ankles. Cue your child to use her breath to relax into the pose. One day she might find her head is connecting with her knees *and* her hands are comfortably looping around her feet.

Modifications

For tight teens: Loop a yoga strap around the foot of the extended leg and, sitting up tall, gently pull on the strap, leaning the torso forward until a comfortable stretch is felt.

Variations

REVOLVED HEAD TO KNEE (additional benefit of a twist)

Simple Steps for Kids

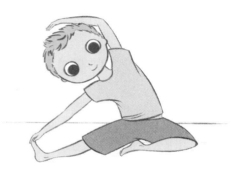

revolved head to knee

- Follow the first two steps in Head to Knee Pose on page 36.

- Do not rotate the torso to align with the extended leg; remain facing forward.

- Nestle your right elbow and forearm along the inseam of the right leg.

- *Inhale:* Lengthen the left arm up and over, reaching it past your head.

- *Exhale:* Slide the right arm along the floor toward your foot; keep reaching your left arm over your head and body toward the right foot.

- Repeat on the left side.

» See this pose in a lesson: energy equalizing (page 170), allergies and colds (page 184), bee (page 199)

Reimagine the Pose!
Strap on Ice Skates, Rollerblades®, or Boots/Shoes • Seated Tree • Giant Nose
Horseback Riding (see strap modification above) • Falling Leaves (revolved variation)

SEATED TWIST

Ardha Matsyendrasana

What Is Seated Twist and How Does It Help?

Seated Twist is a wonderful pose that supports the core and spine. It has the benefits of a hip stretch, twist, and core stabilizer all in one, and it's a lot of fun twisting into a pretzel shape!

 Simple Steps for Kids

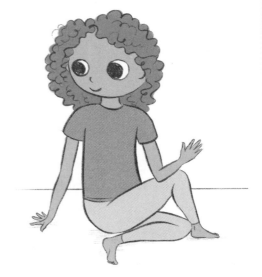

- Begin seated on a yoga mat, legs extended straight out.

- Bend the right knee and draw it in toward your body; lift and place your right foot on the floor outside your left knee. The right knee points up.

- Bend your left knee, tucking your left foot beside your outer right hip. Left knee and thigh should remain in contact with the yoga mat.

- Be sure both hips maintain contact with the floor (if not, see modifications on page 39).

- Place your right hand on the floor beside the right hip and left foot.

- *Inhale:* Lengthen your left arm straight up, reaching it toward the ceiling.

- *Exhale:* Rotate your torso to the right and connect your bent left elbow with the outer right thigh.

- *Inhale:* Lengthen your spine.

- *Exhale:* Maintain spine length and gently twist your torso to the right.

- With each inhale, feel your spine and torso lengthen; use each exhale to gently twist a little deeper into the pose. Use your left elbow as leverage against your right thigh to help you twist, and remember to keep your spine nice and tall.

- Gaze in the direction you are twisting—where the eyes go, the body follows!

- Repeat on other side.

Modifications

Young children with undeveloped motor planning skills (function of the brain to understand, plan, and organize a logical sequence of actions to carry out a task) and bilateral coordination (the ability to move both sides of the body simultaneously in a controlled and coordinated manner) may have trouble creating this pretzel shape. Many teens and tweens will simply be too tight in the hip area to double bind the legs. The following modifications may help:

LEGS: Keep the bottom leg extended straight along the floor, bend the knee of the top leg, and place the foot alongside the knee of the extended leg (ideally, on the outside, but if your teen is super tight, place the foot inside the knee).

ARMS: Tight shoulders may prevent teens from maintaining good alignment when placing the bent elbow on the outer thigh. Cue (i.e., instruct) them to hook the crook of the elbow around the upper shin, or gently place the hand on the outer thigh and use it as leverage to gently ease into the twist.

Variation

SEATED SLIDE TWIST

This variation can be practiced seated in a chair. Rest the hands on the thighs and sit up tall by pressing the butt into the chair. *Inhale:* Lengthen your spine. *Exhale:* Maintain the length and gently twist to the right. Slide your right hand toward your right hip and your left hand along the thigh toward your knee, gaze over the right shoulder. *Inhale:* Back through center, lengthening the spine and sliding the hands to neutral (starting) position on the thighs. *Exhale:* Gently twist to the left, sliding the left hand toward the left hip and the right hand toward the knee, gaze over the left shoulder.

>> **See this pose in a lesson:** tech support (page 181), digestive support (page 188), partner (page 206)

Reimagine the Pose!

Pretzel • Hunter • Twisted Knot • Deer • Robot

STANDING POSTURES

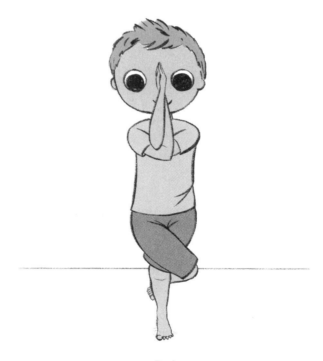

Eagle
(page 71)

MOUNTAIN

Tadasana

What Is Mountain and How Does It Help?

Mountain may appear basic, but it is a mighty strong yoga pose! Practiced correctly, mountain engages every muscle in the body. It is very grounding and stabilizing, as your child presses into the support of the earth beneath her and taps into her quiet inner strength. The benefits of Mountain include core stabilization, postural alignment, and awareness.

 ### Simple Steps for Kids

- Stand with your feet hip-width distance apart.
- Relax your shoulders and rest your arms alongside your torso.
- Gaze straight ahead, chin level with the earth.
- Press your feet evenly into the ground, as if you are trying to push it away; notice how this action engages the muscles in your legs and makes you a little bit taller.
- Slightly tuck your tailbone and notice how this action tightens your tummy (this is engaging your core muscles).
- Rotate your palms to face forward and spread your fingers wide. Notice how this activates the muscles in your arms.
- Hold and breathe, enjoying the strength, stillness, and power of your Mountain.

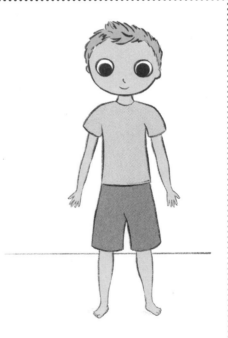

Variations

EXTENDED MOUNTAIN

Reach your arms up to frame your face and rotate your palms inward. Relax the shoulders and press down through your feet; lengthen your body from the feet to fingertips.

EXTENDED MOUNTAIN WITH BABY BACKBEND

Begin in Extended Mountain. ***Inhale:*** Lengthen spine and arms. ***Exhale:*** Maintaining length, gently press the hips forward and lean back, opening your chest toward the ceiling.

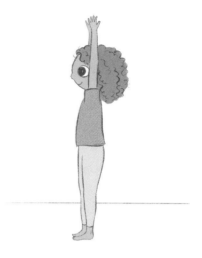

extended mountain

HANDS AT HEART MOUNTAIN

Begin in Mountain. Press your palms together, fingers pointing up and thumbs resting near your heart; relax your shoulders and elbows.

» **See this pose in a lesson:** focus (page 163), good posture and strong core (page 177), allergies and colds (page 184), positive body image (page 191)

Reimagine the Pose!

Name the mountain after your child, for example, "Mount Emily" or "Mount Brendan"

Volcano · Tallest Teepee · Skyscraper · Rocket

STANDING CRESCENT POSE

Indudalasana

What Is Standing Crescent Pose and How Does It Help?

Standing Crescent Pose is a lateral (side) bend that gently stretches and lengthens the spine, torso, and arms. Practicing Standing Crescent Pose stabilizes and strengthens the core and supports spine flexibility.

 ### Simple Steps for Kids

- Begin in Mountain (page 42).
- Sweep arms overhead and connect your palms.
- Clasp fingers and release index fingers, making a steeple.
- Press both feet evenly into the floor. *Inhale:* Lengthen the body from the feet to the tip of your index fingers.
- *Exhale:* Gently bend from your waist to the right. Be sure your arms frame the face and remain aligned with the torso as it lengthens.
- Repeat on the left side.

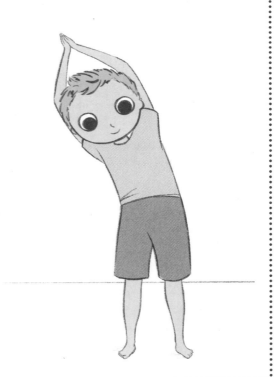

Modifications

Young children may not have the fine motor skills to release the index finger; cue the pose with the palms touching, or try the single-arm variation below.

Variations

SINGLE ARM CRESCENT

Place one hand above the hip, gently gripping the waist. Lengthen the opposite arm up toward the ceiling and breathe in. Breathing out, gently reach the raised arm toward the opposite side of the room, bending the torso with it.

TIP: The hand positioned on the waist acts as a nonverbal cue to lengthen the concave side of the torso instead of crunching or collapsing into it.

SEATED LATERAL BEND

Standing Crescent and Single Arm Crescent poses can be practiced seated in Easy Pose (page 26) or in a chair.

TIPS:

- Lift the chin away from the chest, keeping your shoulders relaxed and rolled back.
- When practicing seated lateral bends, be mindful to keep both hips glued to the mat or seat, and both feet pressing evenly into the floor.
- For a balance challenge, practice lateral bends while holding Tree (page 73) or Low and High Lunge poses (page 53).

» See this pose in a lesson: tech support (page 181), digestive support (page 188), beach adventure (page 202), partner (page 206), teen restorative (page 211)

Reimagine the Pose!

Banana Bend · Boomerang · Hockey Stick · Candy Cane · Kite

STANDING FORWARD FOLD

Uttanasana

What Is Standing Forward Fold and How Does It Help?

Standing Forward Fold is an inversion and a forward bend that stretches the calves and hamstrings, and releases the lower back and hips. This is a great pose if your child does a lot of sitting (in class or at the computer at home). Standing Forward Fold is super relaxing as the upper body dangles over the legs, allowing stress and tension to quite literally drain away.

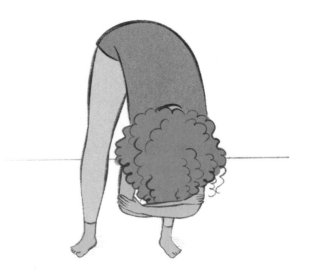

 Simple Steps for Kids

- Begin in Mountain (page 42).

- *Inhale:* Sweep your arms overhead.

- Keep your tummy (core) strong and your spine long.

- *Exhale:* Circle your arms out and hinge from your hips, bending into a forward fold.

- Allow the upper body to dangle over the legs, bending your knees as needed.

- Arms dangle freely, or grip each hand to the opposite elbow.

TIP: If your child has tight hamstrings, which are very common during rapid growth spurts, cue him to bend his knees!

Variations

SEATED IN CHAIR

- Sit squarely on a chair and position your legs the width of the chair in a seated straddle.
- If the feet do not make full contact with the floor, scoot forward in your seat until they do.
- Place your hands on your thighs and straighten your arms, *inhale*, and lengthen your spine and torso.
- Maintaining the length created in your spine, *exhale* and bend from the hips, tracing your hands along the thighs and down your shins toward your feet.
- Tuck in your chin and allow your upper body to simply hang over your legs—arms and hands can dangle, rest on the feet, or grip each hand to the opposite elbow.

>> **See this pose in a lesson:** stress busting (page 167), good posture and strong core (page 177), tech support (page 181), allergies and colds (page 184), beach adventure (page 202)

Reimagine the Pose!

Ragdoll • Empty Coat • Deactivated Robot • Elephant Drinking (clasp hands to make trunk)
Diver (arms up to prepare, forward fold to dive)

GORILLA
Padahastasana

What Is Gorilla and How Does It Help?

Gorilla is an inversion and forward bend that stretches the wrists and shoulders and creates bit of a balance challenge for good measure.

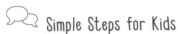 Simple Steps for Kids

- Begin in Standing Forward Fold (page 46).

- Bend both knees deeply.

- Lift one foot at a time and slide your palms, facing up, under your feet. Your fingers should be pointing toward your heels. Lower your feet so your toes rest on or near your wrist creases.

- Once both hands are positioned under the feet, *inhale* fully.

- *Exhale:* Gently straighten both legs.

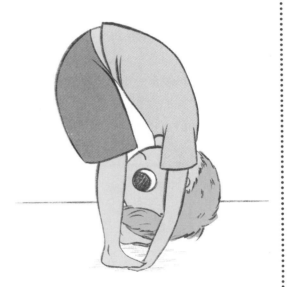

TIP: Deepen this pose by bending the elbows and drawing your torso closer to your legs.

Modifications

YOUNG CHILDREN

The balance challenge posed by placing the hands under the feet may be difficult for young kids. In this case, cue your child to grip her ankles, or stack yoga blocks in front of her and cue her to flip the palms face up and gently press the back of her hands into the blocks.

TWEENS AND TEENS

Kids this age may have trouble with this pose—cue a deep bend in the knees and use yoga blocks for the hands as described above.

No Props? No Problem!

No blocks? No problem. Use the seat of a chair to support the hands; your child may not bend as far forward using a chair, but if his hamstrings are tight, a chair could be just the right height to meet his needs!

» **See this pose in a lesson:** stress busting (page 167)

Reimagine the Pose!

You can be any primate:

Chimpanzee · Monkey · Baboon · Ape · Orangutan

WARRIOR I
Virabhadrasana I

What Is Warrior I and How Does It Help?

Warrior I is a standing hip-stretching pose. Stabilizing and grounding, one truly feels like a strong, unshakeable warrior when holding this pose.

 Simple Steps for Kids

- Begin in Mountain (page 42) and place both hands on the hips.
- Step your left foot toward the back of your yoga mat, positioning it heel down with the toes angled toward the top left corner of your mat.
- Right toes remain pointing straight ahead, perpendicular to the short edge of your mat.
- Bend your right knee to align directly over your right ankle.
- With your hands on your hips, pull the right hip back and the left hip forward so the hips and torso remain square with the front of your mat.
- You may need to adjust the stance of your feet; typically, they should be at least hip-width distance apart, like you are standing on railroad tracks.
- Press both feet evenly into the floor, especially the outer edge and heel of your left foot, which tend to lift in this pose.
- *Inhale:* Sweep your arms overhead, framing your face, reach and lengthen from your hips to your fingertips.
- *Exhale:* Soften your shoulders away from your ears, as your arms continue to lengthen.
- Repeat on the other side.

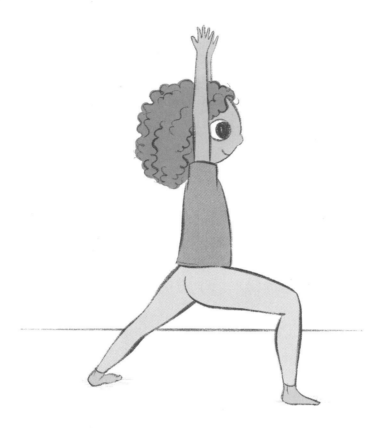

TIP: If your child's back foot does not make contact with the floor, place a folded blanket, towel, or rolled-up yoga mat under it. This will provide the necessary support to experience the correct alignment for this pose.

» **See this pose in a lesson:** focus (page 163), positive body image (page 191), partner (page 206)

Reimagine the Pose!

Touchdown! • Goal Posts • Tall Cactus • Gazelle • Reach for the Stars

CRESCENT LUNGE

Anjaneyasana

What Is Crescent Lunge and How Does It Help?

Crescent Lunge is a hip-stretching *and* back-bending pose with the additional benefit of a balance challenge.

 Simple Steps for Kids

- Begin in Warrior I (page 50), but do not lower or angle the left foot when you step back.

- Keep both feet facing forward and tuck the back toes, lifting your left heel away from the mat.

- Press through the back left heel and straighten the back leg.

- The front knee remains bent and aligned over the front ankle.

- *Inhale:* Sweep your arms to frame your face.

- *Exhale:* Lengthen your torso from the waist and lean back into a gentle backbend, arms framing your torso and head as you lean back.

- Repeat on the other side.

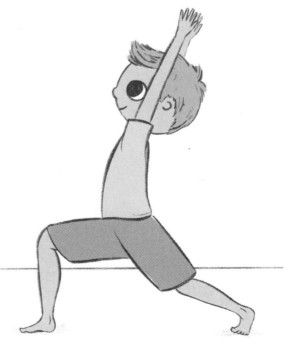

TIP: Strong, active legs make this balance challenge much easier. The following cues will help your child align and keep her balance in this pose:

- "Imagine your front knee and back heel lengthening away from each other."

- "Try not to bend the back knee [unless practicing the Low Lunge variation], keep the leg long and active."

- "Don't forget to breathe—all balancing poses require strong mental focus as much as they do physical strength. Your breath will help keep you focused."

Variations

HIGH LUNGE

Maintain the lunge as outlined above, but keep your arms reaching upward and the shoulders aligned with the hips, as in Warrior I (no backbend).

LOW LUNGE

Drop the back knee to rest on your yoga mat. You have the option to keep the back toes tucked or untucked with the top of the foot on the mat. You can also keep the arms reaching up and the shoulders aligned with your hips (Warrior I arms), or to gently bend back into low Crescent Lunge.

TWISTING LUNGE (additional benefits of a twist and core stabilizer)

- Begin in High or Low Lunge (right side) with your arms extended straight up.

- **Inhale:** Connect your palms.

- **Exhale:** Draw your hands down to the center of your chest.

- **Inhale:** Lengthen the spine—imagine lifting your torso up out of your waist.

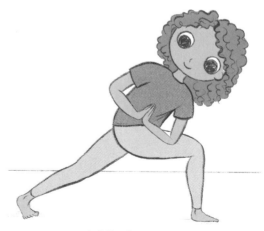

twisting lunge

(pose instructions continue on following page)

- *Exhale:* Maintain this length and gently rotate your torso to the right. Hook your left elbow on the outside of the right thigh.

- Hold and breathe. Lengthen the spine on each inhale and use your left elbow as a lever to gently deepen your twist with each exhale.

- Repeat on the left side.

>> **See this pose in a lesson:** positive body image (page 191), beach adventure (page 202)

Reimagine the Pose!

Dancing Moon • Lunging Lizard • Giant Wave • Around the World • Shield (hook thumbs on both hands and fan fingers before reaching them up and back like a protective shield)

WARRIOR II

Virabhadrasana II

What Is Warrior II and How Does It Help?

Warrior II is a hip-stretching pose and core stabilizer. It builds upper-body strength and inspires kids to be strong, calm, and fierce . . . just like a warrior.

 ## Simple Steps for Kids

- Begin on the right side in Warrior I (page 50) or High Lunge (page 53).

- *Inhale:* Lengthen arms toward the ceiling.

- *Exhale:* Open your arms, reaching them from one end of your mat to the other. At the same time, rotate your left (back) foot so the toes face the long edge of your yoga mat.

- Your front knee remains bent and aligned with the front ankle—glance down and make sure your knee is not rotating inward; if it is, move it toward the right side of your mat so you can see your big toe.

- You may also need to shuffle the feet so your front foot aligns with either the arch or heel of your back foot.

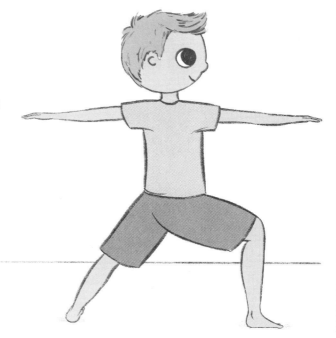

- Keep your arms strong and hands reaching away from each other, as if you are in a tug-of-war; keep your shoulders relaxed. Gaze over your front hand like a brave warrior keeping watch over the horizon.
- Repeat on the other side.

Variations

REVERSE WARRIOR

- Begin in Warrior II.
- Flip the front palm to face the ceiling. *Inhale.*
- *Exhale:* Lean your torso back, reaching your front hand up and overhead toward the back of the room, and resting your back hand on the back leg. Gaze toward the top hand.

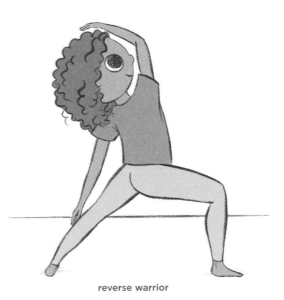

reverse warrior

>> **See this pose in a lesson:** focus (page 163), positive body image (page 191), beach adventure (page 202), partner (page 206)

Reimagine the Pose!

Archer • Surfer • Snowboarder • Skateboarder • Hurdle Jumper (Reverse Warrior)

TRIANGLE

Trikonasana

What Is Triangle and How Does It Help?

Triangle is a hip-stretching and core-stabilizing pose. It stretches the legs, arms, and torso, and can be a bit of a balance challenge, too.

 ## Simple Steps for Kids

- Begin in Warrior II (page 55).

- Straighten the front knee so both legs are straight, forming a triangle shape.

- *Inhale:* Slightly shift the left hip toward the back end of your yoga mat.

- *Exhale:* Reach your right fingertips as far forward as they will go, until you can't reach any farther. Lengthen the arms away from each other (as in Warrior II) and tip your torso so it is parallel with the floor. Reach your right hand toward your right shin or ankle, and your left hand toward the ceiling.

- Use your core muscles to hold your torso parallel with the floor. Gaze toward the top hand; if this is not comfortable or throws off your balance, gaze at the front toes.

- To exit Triangle, press the feet into the floor as if you were trying to push the floor away from you, use the action of pressing down to float your torso back to an upright position.

- Repeat on the left side.

TIP:

- Make sure your child is lengthening both sides of her torso. The tendency is to lean or collapse the side facing the floor, crunching the spine and abdomen. If she is doing this, a block can be helpful: place a block on the inside of the forward leg and adjust it to the required height; rest the front hand on the block instead of the shin or ankle.

- Cue your child to engage his core to hold his body in this position, instead of collapsing his weight into the bottom hand or prop.

» See this pose in a lesson:
focus (page 163), positive body image
(page 191), shape (page 196), bee
(page 199), beach adventure (page 202),
partner (page 206)

Reimagine the Pose!
Teapot • Swimming Starfish • Pyramid
Sail Boat • Ninja Star

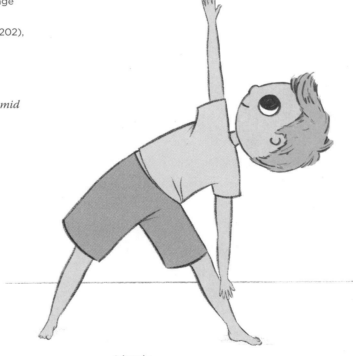

triangle

WIDE LEG FORWARD FOLD

Prasarita Padottanasana

What Is Wide Leg Forward Fold and How Does It Help?

Wide Leg Forward Fold is a magnificent stretch for the hips, legs, and inner thighs that delivers all of the benefits of a forward bend and inversion.

 Simple Steps for Kids

- Face the long edge of your yoga mat and step your feet into a wide stance.
- Reach your arms away from each other at shoulder height, palms down, and shoulders relaxed, making a star shape with your body.
- Adjust your feet to align with the wrists, parallel with the short edges of your yoga mat.
- *Inhale:* Gaze up to the ceiling. Imagine lifting your upper body away from your waist as you lengthen the spine and torso.
- *Exhale:* Maintain length and hinge forward from the hips, stopping halfway with your torso parallel to the floor (like a bird flying over a lake, looking for fish).
- *Inhale:* Realign and lengthen your torso and spine.
- *Exhale:* Maintain that length and fold all the way forward.
- Legs remain straight and strong. Release your arms, connecting your hands to the feet, ankles, or shins.

Modifications

Cue slight-moderate bend in the knees for tight teens as needed, or practice the seated version (on page 60) using props for support. Young children may have a very difficult time balancing. Offer the seated version for toddlers.

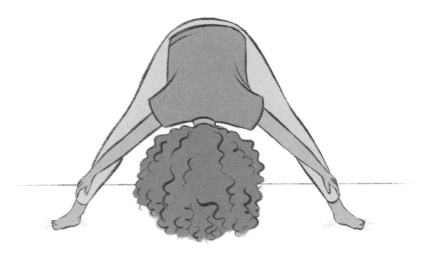

wide leg forward fold

Variations

SEATED WIDE LEG FORWARD FOLD

- Sit on a yoga mat, straddling the legs as wide as you comfortably can.

- Flex your toes toward your body.

- *Inhale:* Reach your arms out wide at shoulder height; lengthen your spine and torso.

- *Exhale:* Keep your core strong and maintain length in your spine, hinge from the hips and reach for the toes as you fold forward.

WIDE LEG TWIST (standing or seated)

- Begin in standing or seated wide leg position.

- *Inhale:* Lengthen the spine and arms—torso parallel to the floor if you're standing and upright if you're sitting.

- *Exhale:* Fold forward and reach the right hand toward the left foot.

- *Inhale:* Center—sit upright if seated, torso parallel to floor if standing.

- *Exhale:* Fold forward, crossing left hand to right foot.

Modifications

If your child has tight hamstrings, cue him to bend his knees or place a soft prop such as a rolled towel under his knees for support. If folding forward is too intense—many tight teens will find this challenging—make this pose restorative by stacking pillows or placing an exercise ball in front of the torso. Relax the upper body and arms over the props and cue slow, full breaths to ease into the stretch.

No Props? No Problem!

If you don't have pillows or an exercise ball, place a chair in front of your child, and cue him to stack his forearms on the seat and gently lean forward, resting his head on his hands.

>> **See this pose in a lesson:** allergies and colds (page 184), shape (page 196), beach adventure (page 202), partner (page 206), teen restorative (page 211)

Reimagine the Pose!

Vulture · Pterodactyl · Goalie · Fallen Snowflake · Clamshell

WARRIOR III

Virabhadrasana III

What Is Warrior III and How Does It Help?

Warrior III is a balancing pose that improves balance skills and core strength. When practiced correctly, the entire body is flexed, strong, and aligned, like a brave warrior's. This is a great pose for overall conditioning, strength, and focus.

 Simple Steps for Kids

- Begin standing in the middle of your yoga mat, facing the short end.
- Step your right foot one or two steps forward, maintaining a hip-width distance from the left foot.
- Reach your arms toward the ceiling, framing your face.
- Turn your palms to face inward, maintaining a shoulder-width space between the hands.
- Lift the left foot away from the mat and point the left toe. Slowly and mindfully tip your body forward, keeping the arms and left leg extended the entire time.
- Stop once your face and torso are parallel to the floor.
- Flex the toes of the extended left leg toward your body, and keep reaching your fingertips forward. Dial the pinkie toe down so that your toes point to the floor, squaring the hips to align correctly.
- Your body should be in a T shape.
- Imagine lengthening from the sole of the back foot to your fingertips with each inhale. Maintain that length and strength as you press your standing foot into the support of the floor, keeping that leg equally strong and engaged with each exhale.
- Repeat on the left side.

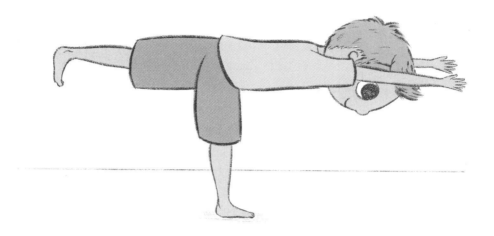

Modifications

YOUNG CHILDREN: Balancing poses can be really challenging for young children, and in a group setting, when one child falls (even unintentionally), it can create a domino effect—the kids break focus, intentionally flopping to the floor and becoming silly. Set kids up for success with the following modifications for Warrior III:

- PARTNERS: Face each other and link hands around your partner's wrists, so you are holding each other's wrists. Step back until your arms extend to full length at shoulder height. Take turns supporting each other tipping forward into Warrior III. Now work together to practice at the same time, supporting each other in a double Warrior III.

- WALL: Align a yoga mat perpendicular to a blank wall (i.e., no shelving, artwork etc.). Place both palms on the wall at shoulder height and walk your feet back until the arms are fully extended. Press the palms into the wall and lift one leg back at a time, tipping the upper body forward as each leg lifts; elbows may bend as you lean forward. Eventually, as you become accustomed to standing on one leg, practicing correct alignment and engagement of the lifted and standing leg, you can move away from the wall and practice Warrior III as described on page 62.

- CHAIR: Place a chair at the top end of the yoga mat (be sure all four legs are on the mat to prevent the chair from slipping). The backrest should be facing you, and the seat of the chair facing out. Stand behind the back of the chair, facing forward. Take a few steps back to allow space for your body, and rest the pinkie finger side of each hand on the back of the chair with the palms facing each other, like you are giving the chair a karate chop. Walk back as far as you can; lengthen your torso and rest your head between your extended arms. Slowly lift and extend one leg at a time, experiencing Warrior III on each side. As you become confident, try lifting your hands away from the chair.

TEENS: Rapid growth spurts and hormonal fluctuations make balance tricky for teens. Offer the same modifications as those for young children above. The following cues and props may also help your teen succeed at Warrior III.

- The more engaged the muscles in the body are, the easier it is to hold the body in a balancing pose; if a part of the body is not engaged, it acts like a dead weight, weighing down the rest of the body.

- Flex the toes of the extended leg toward the face and imagine pressing the sole of that foot into an imaginary wall behind you, push into that imaginary wall as firmly as the grounded foot is pushing into the yoga mat.

- Place a yoga block between the palms and squeeze it, this will help engage the arm muscles.

- Breathe! Use your breath to maintain focus and control when faced with a challenge!

Variations

AIRPLANE POSE

Instead of reaching the arms forward in Warrior III, sweep them back alongside the torso with the palms facing down, like the wings of an airplane. In addition to the benefits of Warrior III, this variation adds a slight backbend to the upper body and gently expands the chest.

» **See this pose in a lesson:** focus (page 163), partner (page 206)

Reimagine the Pose!

Flying Witch ▪ Letter T *▪ Balancing Beam ▪ Airplane*

Magician's Cape (airplane variation)

HALF-MOON

Ardha Chandrasana

What Is Half-Moon and How Does It Help?

Half-Moon is a balancing pose with the additional benefits of a hip stretch and core stabilizer.

 ## Simple Steps for Kids

- Begin in Warrior II (right side, page 55).
- Reach your right hand forward, past your right knee, and place the right fingertips on the floor a few inches forward of your right pinkie toe.
- Lift your left foot off the floor and straighten the right (standing) leg.
- Lengthen your lifted leg and flex the toes, making it as strong and engaged as the standing leg.
- Reach your left arm toward the ceiling—similar to Warrior II, where the arms and hands lengthen away from each other.
- Try to place as little weight as possible in the fingertips resting on the floor.
- Repeat on other side.

Modifications

Place a yoga block on the floor just outside and in front of the forward foot. Adjust the height of the block to meet your child's needs.

No Props? No Problem!

No yoga block? Use a stack of books or the seat of a chair.

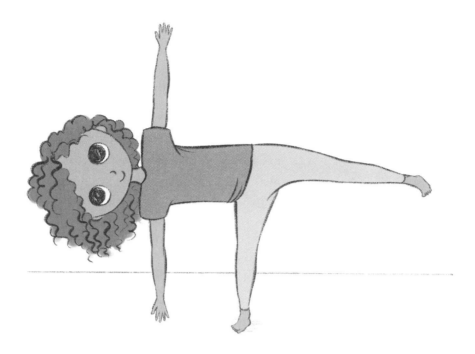

TIP: Help your child strengthen and activate his entire body with the following cues:

- Lengthen from the sole of the lifted leg through the crown of the head.
- Imagine pressing the sole of the foot of the lifted leg into an imaginary wall behind you.
- Push away from the floor with the standing leg.
- Lengthen the fingertips of each hand—imagine energy flowing out of them.
- Lengthen in all directions—imagine energy shooting out of each foot, the fingertips, and the crown of your head.

>> **See this pose in a lesson:** positive body image (page 191)

Reimagine the Pose!

Shooting Star • *Waxing and Waning Moon* • *Flying Saucer* • *Frozen Cartwheel* • *Carnival Ride*

CHAIR POSE

Utkatasana

What Is Chair Pose and How Does It Help?

Chair Pose is often called Awkward Pose because this balancing, core-stabilizing, hip-stretching yoga pose really can feel a little awkward—like sitting in a chair that vanishes just as you are about to connect with the seat. Luckily, we have strong yoga bodies to hold us in place so we don't fall!

Simple Steps for Kids

- Begin in Mountain (page 42).

- *Inhale:* Sweep your arms to frame your face and reach for the ceiling. Relax your shoulders down your back and away from your ears—your shoulders are not earrings!

- *Exhale:* Bend the knees and sit your hips back, as though you are about to sit on an invisible chair.

- Maintain alignment of feet, knees, and legs at hip-width distance.

- Lengthen your body from the hips to the fingertips with each inhale, and drop your butt a little lower with each exhale.

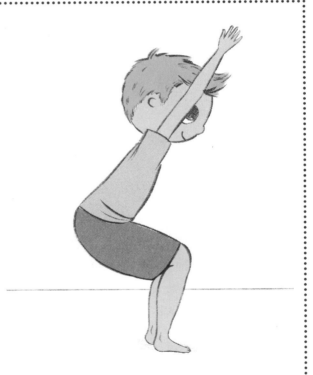

TIP: If your child has trouble maintaining feet and knees at hip-width distance in this pose, place a yoga block between his knees to maintain correct alignment.

Variations

BALANCING CHAIR (additional balance challenge and stretch for the quadriceps and ankles)

- Begin in Chair Pose.
- Connect your palms and lower your hands to your heart center. Press the palms into each other—this helps your body find its center of balance in what is called the midline—the middle part of the body, if you were to split it lengthwise.
- Carefully lift your heels, rising up on your tippy-toes.
- Breathe steadily as you find your balance.
- Lift your heels and check your alignment with each inhale. Use each exhale to slowly and mindfully lower your butt.
- Stay high on your tippy-toes and see how low you can go. Maintain a long spine and balance on your toes without resting your butt on your heels!
- *Inhale:* Straighten your legs with control; remain high on your toes if you can.
- *Exhale:* Lower your heels back to the floor.

TWISTING CHAIR (additional benefits of a twisting pose)

- Begin in Chair Pose, palms touching and resting in front of your heart.
- *Inhale:* Lengthen your spine and torso.
- *Exhale:* Twist right, hooking your left elbow on the outside of your right thigh.

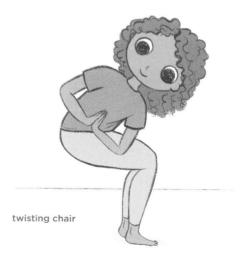

twisting chair

(pose instructions continue on following page)

- Pull your left hip back and right hip forward to maintain alignment of knees and hips with the front of the yoga mat.
- Press the palms into each other and breathe—imagine your spine lengthening on each inhale, maintaining that length as you twist a little deeper with each exhale.
- *Inhale* to unwind. Use your *exhale* to settle back into Chair Pose, facing forward.
- Repeat on other side.

>> **See this pose in a lesson:** stress busting (page 167), positive body image (page 191), partner (page 206)

Reimagine the Pose!

King or Queen on Throne • Baseball Player (Batter up!)
Invisible Chair • Big Dipper • Skier

EAGLE

Garudasana

What Is Eagle and How Does It Help?

Eagle is a challenging yoga pose with multiple benefits. Considered a twist, balance, and hip-stretching posture, it also stretches the shoulders and strengthens the core muscles. Of course, when something is super challenging, like Eagle, focus is the key to success.

 Simple Steps for Kids

* see page 41 for pose illustration

- Begin in Mountain (page 42).

- *Inhale:* Sweep arms overhead to frame your face.

- *Exhale:* Circle arms out and down, crossing them at the elbows, right elbow under left to begin.

- Snake your forearms and hands around each other until the palms connect (this can be tricky; if your child's palms do not connect, see suggested modifications on page 72).

- *Inhale:* Lift elbows to shoulder height.

- *Exhale:* Press the forearms away from your face and gently squeeze the shoulder blades together.

MAINTAIN THIS ALIGNMENT IN THE UPPER BODY AS YOU COMPLETE THE FOLLOWING STEPS:

- *Inhale. Exhale.* Drop your hips back as if you were moving into Chair Pose.

- Lift your right leg up, crossing it over your left leg just above the knee and wrap the lower leg around the calf of your left leg, like a twisted rope (this can be tricky; see modifications on page 72 for help).

- Check that the knees, elbows, feet, and hands remain aligned along the midline of your body; this helps maintain safe alignment of the joints and center of balance.
- Don't forget to breathe! Focus will help you balance and hold Eagle.
- Repeat on the left side.

Modifications

Young children, tweens, and teens who are super tight will find Eagle super challenging. Try the following arm and leg variations, offering the combination that works best for your child:

ARMS

- Cross arms at elbows and rest hands on shoulders.

or

- Cross and bend elbows, align forearms and backs of hands to touch.

LEGS

- Practice arms only if balance is too challenging.
- Cue Chair Pose with Eagle arms (apply above modifications for arms as needed).
- Cross the top leg over, placing the toes on the floor like a kickstand to balance.
- Place the foot of the top leg on a yoga block set up on the inside of the standing leg (it can be moved to the outside of the standing leg as your child becomes comfortable balancing on one leg).

» **See this pose in a lesson:** stress busting (page 167), tech support (page 181), beach adventure (page 202)

Reimagine the Pose!

Stork • Tornado • Licorice Rope • Spiral Shell • Whirlwind

TREE POSE
Vriksasana

What Is Tree Pose and How Does It Help?

Tree Pose is a balancing and hip-opening pose that captures the imagination as much as it engages the core and sharpens focus.

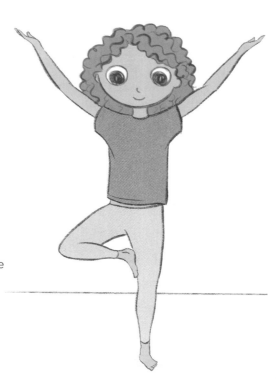

💬 Simple Steps for Kids

- Begin in Mountain (page 42).

- Connect your palms at your heart area; press the palms together to find your center of balance.

- Press both feet into the floor. Imagine growing strong roots, deep into the earth beneath you.

- Lift your right foot and turn your knee outward. Prop the sole of your right foot against your left inner ankle. Toes remain tucked like a kickstand to help with stability.

- Shift your weight into your left foot. Imagine the left leg and torso are the trunk of a big, strong tree.

- Challenge yourself by sliding your right foot along the inside of your leg to rest against the inner calf. Press the sole of your foot into the calf and the calf back into the foot—just like pressing your palms together. This helps to maintain the center of balance along the midline.

- Stay here exploring this version of Tree, or, if you feel stable, slide the foot to the inner thigh, above the knee.

- *Inhale:* Reach the palms overhead. *Exhale:* Open the arms and hands wide, like branches. Relax your shoulders.

- Breathe. Count how many breaths you can hold in Tree Pose standing on this leg.

- Repeat on the other side.

Modifications

Is your child having trouble balancing in Tree? Try the following cues and modifications:

- BUILD A FOREST: Stand side by side and connect palm to palm with the person next to you (this is great for siblings or small groups to work together and support one another). Press into one another's palms (branches) for support and begin to work on lifting the leg for balance.

- WALL: Stand with the back against a wall for support or perpendicular to a wall and place one hand on the wall for stability.

- BLOCK: Acclimate to the hip-opening stretch before adding the balance challenge by placing the lifted foot on a yoga block.

- FEET FIRST: Focus on maintaining balance and stability in the legs before growing branches. Think of strong and resilient winter trees; you don't need big leaf-filled branches to be an awesome tree!

- BREATHE! Trees make oxygen; if you are in Tree Pose, it is super important to breathe—and focusing on your breath will make it much easier to balance.

Trees are unique, just like you—even the same type of tree can look very different from others in the garden. Your tree is perfect exactly how it is; it may look different than your friend's or sibling's tree, and that's okay.

Caution!

Never place the lifted foot on the knee joint—lateral pressure can cause joint strain and injury. Be sure your child places her foot above or below the knee.

» **See this pose in a lesson:** focus (page 163), positive body image (page 191), beach adventure (page 202), partner (page 206)

Reimagine the Pose!

Beach Umbrella • Floating Ghost • Sculpture • Water Fountain

Ask your child what type of tree she is (Apple, Oak, Cherry Blossom, etc.)

KING OF THE DANCERS
Natarajasana

What Is King of the Dancers and How Does It Help?

King of the Dancers could very well be called king of the yoga poses, as it really packs a punch in terms of benefits. The pose is an energizing backbend, balancing, and hip-stretching pose that expands the chest, stretches the shoulders and quadriceps, and lengthens the spine. It requires a lot of focus to maintain King of the Dancers, making it a great pose to hone meditation skills. Let's dance!

 Simple Steps for Kids

- Begin in Mountain (page 42).
- Bend your right knee and bring your right foot toward your butt.
- Rotate your right palm to face away from your body with the thumb pointing behind you. Reach back and grip the inner arch of your right foot with your right hand.
- Align your knees and press down into your left foot for stability.
- *Inhale:* Reach your left arm past your ear toward the ceiling.
- *Exhale:* Flex your right foot; feel it press into the hand holding it.
- Begin to dance: With each inhale, reach your left hand forward, and with each exhale, lift and kick your right foot behind you. Your torso will naturally begin to tilt forward as the foot kicks back, creating a bow shape with your body.
- Reverse the above steps to gracefully exit the pose. Switch sides.

TIP: It's very important to maintain the subtle movement of reaching with each inhale and kicking with each exhale—this will keep your child balanced and focused!

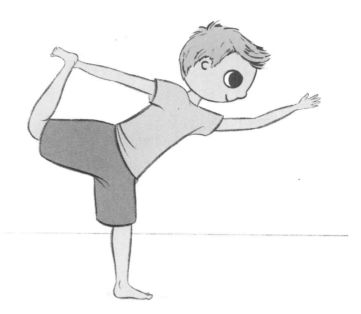

Modifications

WALL: Practice the pose facing a wall. Rest the palm of the raised arm against the wall and work on the quad stretch, balance, and kicking the lifted foot back and up.

PARTNER UP: Face your partner, connecting the palms of your forward hands. Press into each other's palms for support as you work on balance and lifting and kicking the foot.

PRACTICE IN STAGES: Master one stage at a time before moving to the next.

- **STAGE ONE:** Stand on one leg and hold the lifted foot. (This is a good quad stretch and a great way to explore balance, alignment, and focus.)

- **STAGE TWO:** Reach arm up and forward.

- **STAGE THREE:** Kick the lifted foot back and reach the raised arm forward. Notice how the equal and opposite movement of reaching and kicking helps you to maintain balance.

» **See this pose in a lesson:** focus (page 163), partner (page 206)

Reimagine the Pose!

Figure Skater • Dancing Queen (or King) • Dinosaur • Giraffe • Construction Crane

SQUAT

Malasana

What Is Squat and How Does It Help?

A wonderful release for the lower back and hips, Squat is so much more than a simple hip-stretching pose; it stabilizes and strengthens the core, improves balance, and supports digestive health.

Simple Steps for Kids

- Stand with your feet as wide as your yoga mat, toes pointed out and heels in.

- Bring your palms together at the center of your chest. Relax your shoulders.

- *Inhale. Exhale:* Lower your hips toward the floor—keep your spine and torso as tall and upright as you can!

- Nestle your elbows against your inner thighs, and gently press against the thighs to open the knees.

- Lengthen your tailbone toward the floor and your crown toward the ceiling.

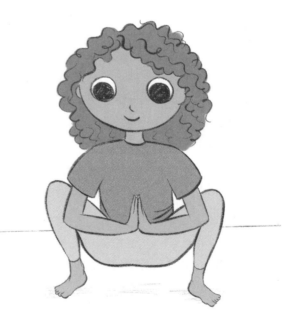

TIPS:

ALIGNMENT: If your child's heels do not make contact with the floor, cue her to widen her stance. If that doesn't help, bring the floor to her with this simple trick: Place a rolled or folded yoga mat under her heels.

BALANCE TIP: To support hip opening and upper body alignment without the balance challenge, place a yoga block under your child's hips so she is sitting on the block while in Squat. Once she builds strength and confidence, remove the block and work on balance.

» **See this pose in a lesson:** digestive support (page 188)

Reimagine the Pose!
Duck • Campfire Crouch • Frog on a Lily Pad • Sumo Wrestler
Spaceship Launchpad

PRONE POSTURES

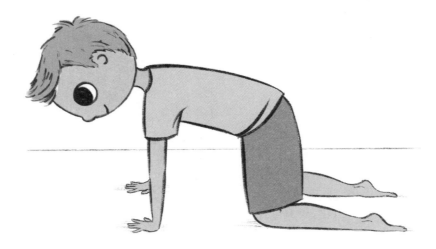

Table
(following page)

TABLE

Bharmanasana

What Is Table and How Does It Help?

Table is a stabilizing and grounding pose that supports alignment in the torso. It is commonly used to transition into Downward Facing Dog, or to and from standing and prone postures. Table strengthens the wrists, upper body, and core while aligning and lengthening the spine.

 Simple Steps for Kids

* see previous page for pose illustration

- Begin on your hands and knees.

- Align your knees directly below your hips. Shins and feet rest along the floor, at a right angle to the knees.

- Tuck your toes to gently stretch the soles of your feet, or flip your feet so the tops rest on the floor, soles face the ceiling. Gently press your shins and feet into the floor.

- Align your hands directly under your shoulders. Spread your fingers wide and press your hands evenly into the floor.

- Arms should be straight. Slightly hug your shoulders together behind your back and draw them away from your ears.

- Gaze a few inches in front of your hands to maintain a neutral position in the cervical spine (the part of your spine that supports your neck).

- Hold and breathe; *inhale:* Lengthen your tailbone and crown away from one another.

- *Exhale:* Relax into the space and alignment you are creating in your body.

Variations

LEG LIFTS

Lift one leg at a time from Table position, bending the knee and raising the leg in the air. Be mindful to keep both hips facing down, square with the floor. Switch legs.

REVERSE TABLE:

Flip your Table so your body faces up, palms down, fingers pointing to the feet. Press into the hands and feet to lift your body, aligning your belly with your hips and shoulders. Don't let your butt sag toward the floor.

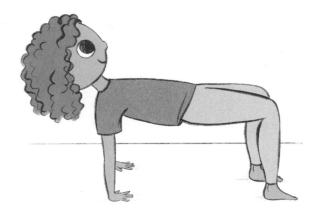

reverse table

» See this pose in a lesson: good posture and strong core (page 177), shape (page 196), bee (page 199), beach adventure (page 202), teen restorative (page 211)

Reimagine the Pose!

Square • Picnic Table • Bee Stinger (lift leg, point toe)

Rectangle (Reverse Table) • Crab (Reverse Table)

CAT-COW
Marjaryasana-Bitilasana

What Is Cat-Cow and How Does It Help?

Cat-Cow is a yoga stretch where two poses (Cat and Cow) are cued to flow back and forth between each other. A gentle warm-up to loosen kinks or tight spots in the body before practicing yoga, Cat-Cow provides the benefits of a forward bend, backbend, hip stretch, and mild inversion all in one simple practice.

Simple Steps for Kids

- Begin in Table (page 81).

- *Inhale:* Drop your belly toward the floor. Lengthen your tailbone and crown away from each other, creating a beautiful bow shape with your spine. Keep your arms and legs strong and pressing into the floor. This is Cow Pose.

- *Exhale:* Tuck in your chin and tailbone and arch your spine like a cat. Lengthen your spine in the opposite direction. Gaze between your thighs to maintain length in your cervical spine (neck). This is Cat Pose.

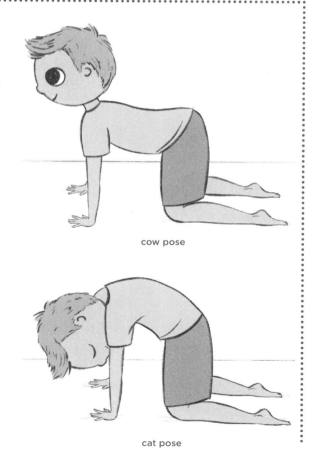

cow pose

cat pose

- Move back and forth between Cat and Cow poses, linking your body's movement to your breath. Use your whole inhale to move into Cow, arriving in the full expression of Cow at the top of your inhale. Begin your exhale and start to move into Cat, arriving in the full expression at the bottom of the exhale.

Variations

SEATED CAT-COW

- Sit in a chair, feet square on the floor in front of you. Do not lean into the support of the chair; instead press into the seat with your butt and feel your spine float to a naturally erect position, or sit on the floor in Easy Pose.

- Rest your hands on your knees or thighs.

- *Inhale:* Gently pull on the knees to expand your chest and squeeze the shoulders together— imagine lengthening your tailbone and crown away from each other as your spine makes a bow shape. This is Seated Cow.

- *Exhale:* Tuck your tailbone and chin and pull your belly button in, curling (but still lengthening!) your spine in the opposite direction. This is Seated Cat.

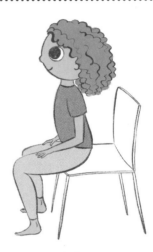

seated cow

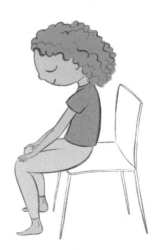

seated cat

DANCING LION

- Begin in Table and *inhale* to center yourself.

- *Exhale:* Draw a circle with your hips, moving to the right back corner of the yoga mat and around to the left.

- *Inhale:* Continue to circle your hips forward of the knees (your shoulders will also come forward of the wrists) and to the right.

- Make circles with your body—big or small; it's your lion and he can dance in a way that feels good to him! Switch directions to balance out your lion.

» **See this pose in a lesson:** warming up (page 142), stress busting (page 167), good posture and strong core (page 177), tech support (page 181), digestive support (page 188), teen restorative (page 211)

Reimagine the Pose!

Any big cat—Panther, Lion, Jaguar, Cheetah • Armadillo

Edaphosaurus (curl into Cat to create sail-like fin)

Sagging Bridge (Cow); Solid Bridge (Cat) • Smile (Cow); Frown (Cat)

THREAD THE NEEDLE

Parsva Balasana

What Is Thread the Needle and How Does It Help?

Thread the Needle is a twist, shoulder stretch, and mild inversion—it also gently stretches the feet!

 Simple Steps for Kids

- Begin in Table (page 81) with the toes tucked to stretch the feet and toes.
- *Inhale:* Sweep your right arm out and up toward the ceiling. Follow your hand with your gaze.
- *Exhale:* Sweep the right hand, palm facing up, under your body and through the "loop" created by your left arm and the floor.
- Breathe normally as you nestle your right shoulder on the floor and rest the right side of your head on the floor.
- Support the head and/or shoulder with a folded blanket or towel if needed.
- Hold this pose for several rounds of breath. Gently unwind from the pose, the same way you came in, and return to Table.
- Repeat on the left side.

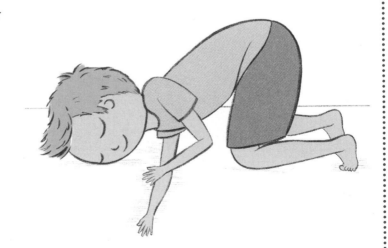

Modifications

If your child is ready for a deeper stretch, try the following: Once positioned in Thread the Needle, sweep the upper arm toward the ceiling, bend at the elbow, and rest the back of the hand on the lower back.

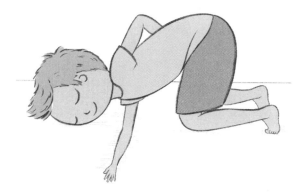

modified thread the needle

» **See this pose in a lesson:** good posture and strong core (page 177), teen restorative (page 211)

Reimagine the Pose!

Tailor · *Spaghetti Noodle* · *Cave Explorer* · *Burrowing Bunny*

Snake (hiding in a cave or under a rock!)

PLANK

Utthita Chaturanga Dandasana

What Is Plank and How Does It Help?

Plank can be a challenging pose. The whole body is strong and engaged when practicing this pose. It is especially helpful for building a strong core and strengthening the upper body and wrists.

 Simple Steps for Kids

- Begin in Table (page 81), hands positioned toward the top of your yoga mat.
- Step one foot at a time toward the back end of the mat, lengthening each leg and tucking the toes so that only your tucked toes and two palms are making contact with the yoga mat.
- Press the floor away with your hands and squeeze your shoulders together behind your back; this will help to engage your upper body.
- Press through your heels to engage your legs so they are straight and strong!
- The action of engaging your arms and legs by pressing equally through the palms and heels supports engagement and strengthening of the core to protect the back from strain or injury in this pose.
- Gaze in front of your palms to maintain a neutral position in the neck.
- Your body should be in one straight line from crown to heels.

Modifications

Plank can be challenging for kids who have yet to develop the strength to safely maintain the pose. If your child's hips or torso sag or lift, cue him to realign. If his hips still scoop or dip, cue him to lower his knees to the floor while holding Plank.

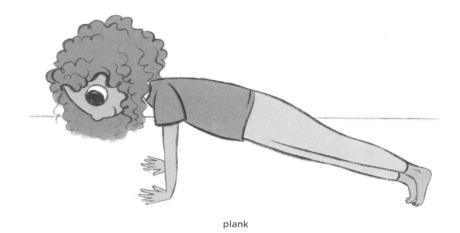

plank

Variations

LOW PUSH-UP (Chaturanga Dandasana)

- *Inhale* in Plank (knees up or down).

- *Exhale:* Slowly bend elbows at a 90-degree angle, hugging them close to the torso; lower your body to hover at the same height as the bent elbows.

- If your knees are lifted, it is important to maintain the same engagement and alignment in Low Push-Up as Plank—with core strong, press evenly into the palms and back through the heels. Breathe!

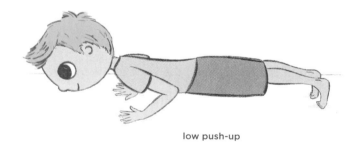

low push-up

SIDE PLANK (additional balance challenge)

- Begin in Plank. Reposition your right palm to the center of your yoga mat.

- Roll to the outer edge of your right foot, turning your body to face the left side of the room.

- Stack your left foot on top of your right (inner edges touching), flex both feet, and press the outer edge of your right foot into the floor. The outer edge of your right foot and palm are the only body parts touching the floor.

- Reach your left arm up toward the ceiling; press the right palm into the floor and lengthen the arms and hands away from each other.

- Lift the outer hip toward the ceiling to prevent sagging in this pose.

- Return to Plank and repeat on the other side.

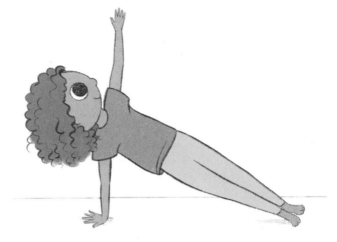

side plank

Modifications

Try these to decrease or increase the challenge in Side Plank:

- For added stability, place the top foot in front of the bottom foot and press the inner edge into the floor.

- Drop the knee of the bottom leg to the floor for additional support.

- For a challenge, bend the knee of the top leg and place your foot on the inseam of the bottom leg, making Tree Pose in Side Plank.

DOLPHIN PLANK

- Begin in Table.

- Bend your elbows and place your forearms and hands on the yoga mat in front of you. Clasp each elbow with the opposite hand (this step is important to align the shoulders and prevent strain or injury).

- Release your grip and—keeping the elbows spaced as measured above—clasp your hands, creating a triangle with the elbows, forearms, and hands.

- Press your forearms and clasped hands into the yoga mat and step one foot at a time to the back end of your yoga mat.

- Lengthen from the crown to the heels, just as you do in regular Plank.

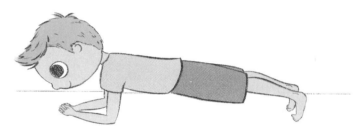

dolphin plank

» See this pose in a lesson: focus (page 163), good posture and strong core (page 177)

Reimagine the Pose!

Alligator/Crocodile ▪ Log ▪ Sword ▪ Pirate's Plank
Magical Mystical Floating Trick

COBRA

Bhujangasana

What Is Cobra and How Does It Help?

Cobra is a backbend that lengthens the spine and strengthens back muscles. It also broadens the chest and shoulders to counter rounded or slumped shoulders.

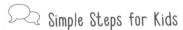 Simple Steps for Kids

- Begin lying on your belly on a yoga mat.

- Place feet together or hip-width distance apart, with the soles facing up.

- Bend your elbows, place your hands, palms down, on the yoga mat and aligned beneath your shoulders. Hug your elbows to your torso so they point up.

- Rest your chin on the yoga mat.

- *Inhale:* Press the tops of your feet, pelvis, and hands into the floor. Squeeze your elbows and shoulder blades toward each other as you broaden your chest. Lengthen your crown away from your tailbone and peel the upper body away from the floor.

- *Exhale* slowly with a "hsss . . ." as you hold Cobra.

- *Inhale:* Lift and lengthen the spine and torso.

- *Exhale:* Slowly lower your body back to the mat.

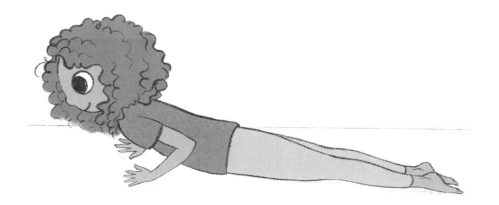

» **See this pose in a lesson:** good posture and strong core (page 177), beach adventure (page 202)

Reimagine the Pose!

Hissing Snake · Hungry Worm · Skateboard Ramp · Otter · Body Surfer

UPWARD FACING DOG

Urdhva Mukha Svanasana

What Is Upward Facing Dog and How Does It Help?

Commonly referred to as "Up Dog," Upward Facing Dog is a backbend and chest-opening pose. A deeper and fuller backbend than Cobra (page 92), it is important to warm up with a few rounds of Cobra before practicing Up Dog.

 Simple Steps for Kids

- Begin in Cobra.

- Shift your palms one handprint back from the shoulders to frame your ribs.

- *Inhale:* Press the palms and tops of your feet into the floor. Feel your spine lengthen (crown and tailbone moving away from each other) as you straighten your arms.

- *Exhale:* Relax your shoulders away from your ears.

- Only the palms and tops of the feet make contact with the mat in Upward Facing Dog.

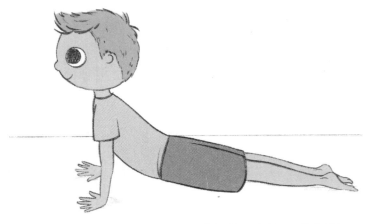

» **See this pose in a lesson:**
good posture and strong core
(page 177)

Reimagine the Pose!
Wave • Roller Coaster
Striking Snake • Howling Wolf
Hockey/Soccer Net

SPHINX

Salamba Bhujangasana

What Is Sphinx and How Does It Help?

Sphinx is a backbend that strengthens the arms and shoulders, lengthens the spine, and broadens the chest.

 Simple Steps for Kids

- Rest on your belly and prop your upper body on your elbows.
- Clasp each elbow with the opposite hand to safely align your shoulders.
- Release your hands and, without moving your elbows, turn your forearms to face forward with your palms down.
- Press into your forearms and lift your chest so your shoulders align with the elbows—hips, legs, and feet remain in contact with the yoga mat.
- Lengthen your spine on each inhale; soften your shoulders with each exhale.

» **See this pose in a lesson:** stress busting (page 167)

Reimagine the Pose!

Egyptian Sphinx • Bask in the Sun
Iguana • Open Window • Sea Lion

DOWNWARD FACING DOG

Adho Mukha Svanasana

What Is Downward Facing Dog and How Does It Help?

Often referred to as "Down Dog," Downward Facing Dog is a forward bend, inversion, and full body stretch. It lengthens and stretches the spine, calves, and hamstrings; builds upper and lower body strength; and releases tension from the lower back and hips. Although it can be challenging at first, Down Dog is often cued as a resting pose during a yoga practice to realign the body and catch the breath before transitioning to another pose.

 Simple Steps for Kids

- Begin in Table (page 81).
- *Inhale:* Tuck your toes so the soles of your feet face behind you.
- *Exhale:* Lift your tailbone toward the ceiling. Straighten your legs and drop your heels toward the floor (it's okay if they don't completely touch the floor).
- Arms and legs are straight, tailbone points up and back—you should look like an upside-down V shape.
- Press into your palms and lengthen your body from hands to hips.
- Press your heels down and lengthen your legs from hips to heels.
- Press your chest toward your thighs.
- Relax your shoulders away from your ears (this is hard to do when you're upside down), and allow your head to rest between your arms.

» **See this pose in a lesson:** energy equalizing (page 170), good posture and strong core (page 177), tech support (page 181), allergies and colds (page 184), positive body image (page 191), partner (page 206)

Reimagine the Pose!

Hill • Artist's Easel • Tunnel

Open Book • Rooftop

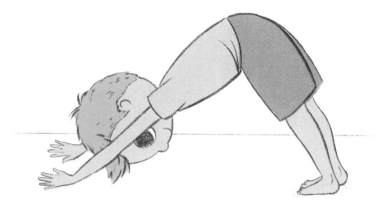

downward facing dog

Variation

PUPPY POSE

- Begin in Table. Keep the knees down, tuck your toes, and press the hips back to hover over your heels.

- Walk your hands forward and straighten your arms.

- Lengthen your spine, from crown to tailbone, as you relax your torso and head between your arms.

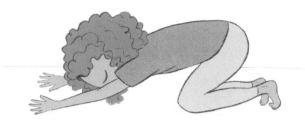

puppy pose

SEATED DOG (seated at desk)

- Push the chair away from the edge of the desk to allow space for your arms and torso.

- Reach your arms forward and rest your palms, face down, on the desk. Remain seated and press your feet evenly into the floor.

- *Inhale*: Press into your palms and lengthen your spine.

- *Exhale:* Hinge from the hips, keep your spine long, and lower your torso and head between your extended arms.

- Keep pressing your palms into the desk. Hold and breathe, enjoying the stretch.

DOLPHIN POSE
Ardha Pincha Mayurasana

What Is Dolphin Pose and How Does It Help?

Dolphin is an upper-body strengthening pose with the added benefits of a forward bend, inversion, and balance challenge.

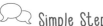 Simple Steps for Kids

- Begin in Table (page 81), toes tucked.

- Bend the elbows and rest your forearms and hands on the yoga mat in front of you. Clasp each elbow with the opposite hand (this step is important to align the shoulders and prevent strain or injury).

- Release your grip and clasp your hands, creating a triangle with the elbows, forearms, and hands.

- *Inhale:* Press your forearms and clasped hands into the yoga mat.

- *Exhale:* Lift your hips toward the ceiling, drop your heels toward the floor— legs straight and spine long, just like in Downward Facing Dog.

- Hold and breathe, working on building upper-body strength in this stage of the pose.

IF YOUR CHILD IS COMFORTABLE IN THIS STAGE OF THE POSE, PROCEED TO THE NEXT STAGE.

- Walk your feet closer to your body, keeping the legs straight! Continue pressing the forearms into the floor and keep the shoulders away from your ears (this is difficult to do when you're upside down!).

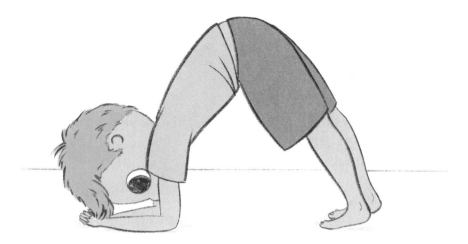

Modifications

Young children tend to place their head on the floor in this pose, straining the neck and risking injury. Cue Baby Dolphin (Dolphin Pose with knees down) for young children.

» **See this pose in a lesson:** good posture and strong core (page 177), beach adventure (page 202)

Reimagine the Pose!

Swimming Dolphin · *Inchworm* · *Tent* · *Drawbridge* · *Scuba Diver*

HALF PIGEON

Eka Pada Raja Kapotasana

What Is Half Pigeon and How Does It Help?

Half Pigeon is a hip-stretching, spine-lengthening forward bend. Best practiced toward the end of a yoga session, when the body and joints have warmed up, some find Half Pigeon challenging, while others find it restorative.

💬 Simple Steps for Kids

- Begin in Downward Facing Dog (page 96).
- *Inhale:* Lengthen the right leg up behind you.
- *Exhale:* Bend the right knee and guide the right leg under your body toward the top of your yoga mat.
- Place the right knee behind the right wrist and the right ankle near the left side of your mat; position the shin so it is parallel with the top of the yoga mat (it may be difficult for your child to position her leg completely parallel, and that's okay—for some, the leg may make the shape of a number 7; for others it may look more like a check mark).
- Lower the hips toward the floor, left leg extending straight back along the mat, untuck your left toes, and rest the top of the foot on the floor.
- Square your shoulders and hips with the front of your yoga mat. You may need to pull the right hip back and left hip forward.
- *Inhale:* Lift and lengthen your spine and torso.
- *Exhale:* Walk your hands forward until your torso rests over your front leg.
- Reverse out of the pose the same way you entered. Repeat on the left side.

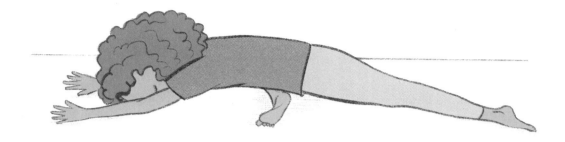

Modifications

Half Pigeon may be really challenging for teens and tweens with tight muscles. Try the following modifications or cue Reclined Pigeon (variation below).

- Focus on stretching the legs and hips: Place the forward leg at the top of the yoga mat, but do not fold forward. Frame the hips with the hands (use yoga blocks if needed), straighten the arms, and breathe.

- If your child's hip is tilting toward the floor, place a folded blanket or pillow under the hip to align her pelvis and square her hips and shoulders to face forward. Give her the option to move into a forward fold.

Variation

RECLINED PIGEON

- Lie on your back on a yoga mat with the knees bent and feet flat on the floor.

- Place feet and knees hip-width distance apart.

- Lift the right foot and place the right ankle across the left thigh, just below the knee, making a figure 4 with the legs.

- Reach your right hand through the loop your right leg is making, and place the left hand around the outer left leg.

- Lift the left foot off the floor. Maintain the figure 4 shape with the right leg.

- Clasp your hands around the back of the left thigh or top of the left shin.

- Rest your upper body on the floor and gently pull the left leg toward the body.

- Reverse to unwind from the pose and repeat on the left side.

» **See this pose in a lesson:** good posture and strong core (page 177), teen restorative (page 211)

Reimagine the Pose!

Plant and Cover Seeds • Lazy Leopard • Snoozing Swan • Needle in a Haystack

Basketball Hoop (Reclined Pigeon)

CROCODILE

Makarasana

What Is Crocodile and How Does It Help?

A gentle and restorative yoga pose, Crocodile is stabilizing and grounding, with the added benefits of a mild backbend to gently expand the shoulders and chest.

 Simple Steps for Kids

- Lie on your belly with your hands stacked at the top of your yoga mat.

- Rest your forehead on top of your stacked hands.

- Relax into the support of your stacked hands and the floor beneath you.

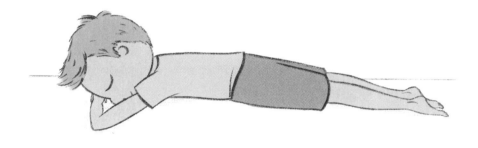

Variation

WINDSHIELD WIPER LEGS

- Bend knees and gently rock the lower legs from side to side, like windshield wipers.

>> See this pose in a lesson: good posture and strong core (page 177), allergies and colds (page 184), teen restorative (page 211)

Reimagine the Pose!

Floating Log • Fallen Tree • Speed Bump • Mermaid's/Merman's Tail (var.) • Synchronized Swimmer (var.)

LOCUST

Shalabasana

What Is Locust and How Does It Help?

Locust is an energizing backbend that stretches the front side of the body and strengthens the back.

 Simple Steps for Kids

- Begin by lying on your belly with your arms resting by your torso, palms down.
- Rest your forehead on the floor.
- *Inhale:* Press your feet and pelvis into the floor. Peel your chest and upper body upward. Lift your arms and reach your fingertips toward the back of your mat, palms remain facing down.
- *Exhale:* Soften your shoulders away from your ears.
- *Inhale:* Lift your legs off the floor and lengthen your whole body from toes to crown. Keep reaching back with the hands.
- *Exhale:* Relax your shoulders and reach your hands back. Continue lifting your legs and chest.
- Try to lift a little higher with each inhale, using each exhale to maintain alignment but softening into the pose.

» See this pose in a lesson: energy equalizing (page 170), good posture and strong core (page 177), positive body image (page 191), beach adventure (page 202)

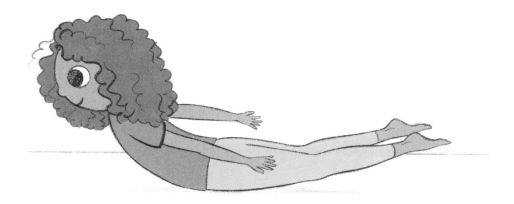

Variation

TAKE FLIGHT

- Reach your arms in front of you—lift your legs and arms from the floor.
- **BILATERAL MOVEMENT:** Reach your arms in front and alternate lifting and lowering the opposite arm and leg. For example, inhale to lift the right arm and left leg, lower on exhale; inhale to lift the left arm and right leg, lower on exhale.

Modifications

Sensitive groin areas do not like this pose! Place a soft pillow, towel, or folded blanket under the groin, or offer your child an alternative backbend, such as Bridge Pose (page 115).

Reimagine the Pose!

Superpower: Flight! · *Flying Snake* · *Swimming Fish* · *Leaping Lizard* · *Shark*

BOW

Dhanurasana

What Is Bow and How Does It Help?

Bow, one of the biggest back-bending poses in yoga, stretches the entire front side of the body: the shoulders, chest, arms, thighs, shins, and feet. Bow is very energizing, as the whole body fires up its muscles to hold the pose.

 Simple Steps for Kids

- Lie on your belly.
- Bend your knees and reach one hand at a time back to grip the outer ankle of each foot.
- Align the knees, hip-width distance apart.
- *Inhale:* Flex the feet and kick them back, lifting knees, chest, and upper body away from the floor.
- *Exhale:* Kick the feet up and back.
- Lift and lengthen the torso on each inhale; kick your feet and shins up and back with each exhale. Feel the strength of your legs gently lift and expand your upper body.
- Visualize your spine as a bow—no crunching! Imagine the tailbone and crown moving away from each other.

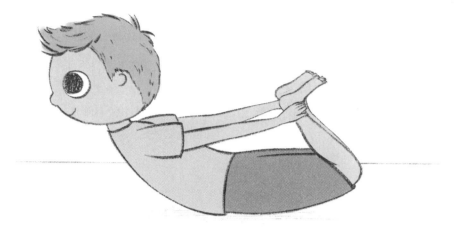

Modifications

If your child finds this pose challenging, practice one side at a time—Half Bow Pose.
If your child can't reach his feet—tight teens may not be able to—use a strap.

»» See this pose in a lesson: energy equalizing (page 170), good posture and strong core (page 177),
positive body image (page 191)

Reimagine the Pose!

Apple • Bucket • Energy Circuit • Flexing Snake • Nest

CAMEL

Ustrasana

What Is Camel and How Does It Help?

Camel is a deep back-bending pose that offers the additional benefits of a hip stretch and core stabilizer. When practiced to its fullest expression, it is considered an inversion.

 Simple Steps for Kids

- Begin standing on your knees, knees spaced hip-width distance apart.
- Place your hands on your lower back, thumbs out and fingers down, like you are sliding your hands into imaginary pockets.
- Relax your shoulders. Squeeze the shoulder blades and elbows toward each other.
- *Inhale:* Lengthen your upper body as you lift it up and away from the waist.
- *Exhale:* Slowly bend back, opening your chest and face toward the ceiling. Keep your hips in line with your knees. Press into your lower back with your hands to move the hips forward and lengthen the lower back.
- On each inhale, lengthen the spine, and on each exhale, see if you can safely and comfortably lean farther back.
- If your heels are within reach, move one hand at a time from the lower back to grip the heel of each foot; fingers grip the inner arches and thumbs on the outside of each foot. Tuck the toes to add height as needed.
- Press the hips forward and imagine the spine lengthening from the tailbone to the crown. Breathe.

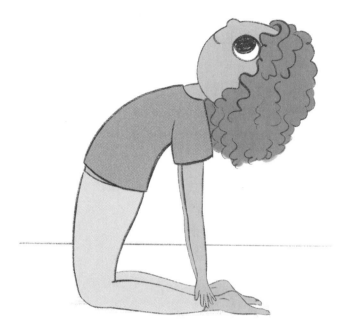

Modifications

- To work on alignment, have your child practice Camel facing a wall. Cue him to press his hips into the wall and maintain that contact as he moves into Camel.

- If you notice your child is crunching his spine, place an exercise ball on the back of his thighs and cue him to lift his body up and over the ball.

❯❯ See this pose in a lesson: energy equalizing (page 170), partner (page 206)

Reimagine the Pose!

Letter D · *Turtle Shell* · *Hippopotamus* · *Thirsty Camel* · *Circle Back*

RABBIT

Sasangasana

What Is Rabbit and How Does It Help?

Rabbit is a restorative forward bend and inversion that stretches the shoulders and releases the lower back and hips. It is often cued following a deep backbend (such as Camel) as a counter stretch.

 ### Simple Steps for Kids

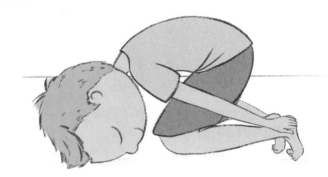

- Begin by sitting on your knees, toes tucked and butt resting on the heels.
- Reach your hands back and grip the heels of each foot, thumbs out, fingers in.
- *Inhale:* Lengthen your torso and spine.
- *Exhale:* Gently fold forward, resting your crown on the floor and forehead against the knees.
- *Inhale:* Lift your hips and extend them toward the ceiling.
- *Exhale:* Straighten your arms and pull on your heels for resistance.
- Be sure not to place pressure or weight on the head or neck; the crown should barely touch the floor.

» **See this pose in a lesson:** energy equalizing (page 170), beach adventure (page 202)

Reimagine the Pose!

Coiled Shell · Groundhog · Seahorse · Yo-yo · Curly Spring

CHILD'S POSE

Balasana

What Is Child's Pose and How Does It Help?

Child's Pose is a restorative forward-bending pose that gently stretches the lower back and hips. It is an ideal pose to take a rest during yoga practice or any time you need to calm and center your mind or body.

 Simple Steps for Kids

- Begin by sitting on your knees with your butt resting on your heels.
- Fold your upper body over your knees, resting your forehead on the floor.
- Reach the arms straight ahead, resting your palms on the floor, and lengthen from your hips to fingertips; or place your arms alongside your torso with the palms facing up near your feet.

Modification

If your child's head does not meet the floor, bring the floor to her: Place a block, bolster, or folded towel under her forehead, or cue her to stack her hands and rest her forehead on them for support.

>> **See this pose in a lesson:** stress busting (page 167), energy equalizing (page 170), chilling out (page 173), good posture and strong core (page 177), allergies and colds (page 184), bee (page 199), beach adventure (page 202), teen restorative (page 211)

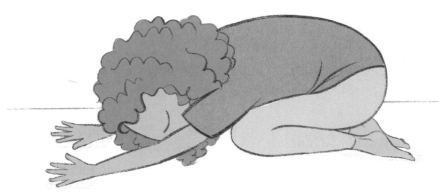

child's pose (arms extended)

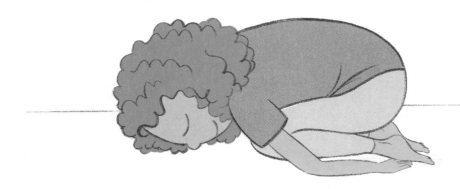

child's pose (arms by side)

Variations

WIDE LEG CHILD'S POSE

- Begin by sitting on your knees.

- Open your knees wide and bring your toes in to touch.

- *Inhale:* Lengthen the torso. *Exhale:* Walk your hands and arms forward, folding the upper body until the torso rests between the knees on the yoga mat.

- Imagine sinking your hips into your heels as you reach your arms forward. Lengthen your arms and body, from hips to your fingertips.

SUPPORTED CHILD'S POSE

- Start in the Wide Leg Child's Pose variation, before folding forward. Position a bolster or pillow between your thighs; it should be vertical on the mat (perpendicular to the body).

- *Inhale:* Lengthen the torso.

- *Exhale:* Slowly lower the torso to rest on the bolster.

- Rest your left ear on the bolster. After a few rounds of breath, switch and face the other direction.

CRESCENT CHILD'S POSE

- Start in regular Child's Pose with the arms extended forward or Wide Leg Child's Pose variation.

- *Inhale:* Lengthen the torso and arms.

- *Exhale:* Walk the hands toward the left corner of your yoga mat to make a crescent shape and stretch the right side of the body. Hold and breathe. Repeat on the other side.

Reimagine the Pose!

Moon Rock ▪ Beehive ▪ Seed ▪ Egg ▪ Sleeping Snake

SUPINE POSTURES

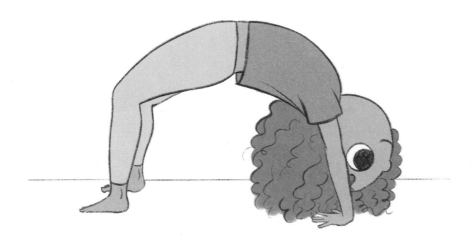

Upward Facing Bow
(page 117)

BRIDGE
Setu Bandhasana

What Is Bridge and How Does It Help?

Bridge is a backbend, hip opener, and mild inversion.

💬 Simple Steps for Kids

- Begin by lying on your back.

- Bend your knees and place your feet on the floor.

- Space knees and feet hip-width distance apart.

- Place your arms alongside your torso with the palms facing down.

- *Inhale:* Press your feet, shoulders, forearms, and palms into the floor as you lift your hips up.

- *Exhale:* Press your feet and arms into the floor to lift the hips higher, forming a bridge shape from shoulders to knees.

- Imagine water flowing underneath your strong bridge.

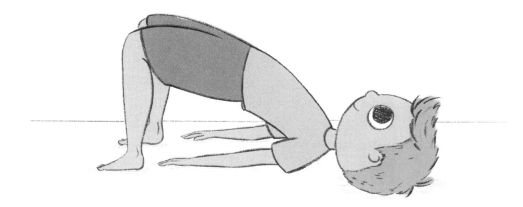

TIP: To maintain leg alignment and engagement, place a yoga block between the knees.

Variations

ROLLING BRIDGE

Move in and out of Bridge, linking movement to breath:

- *Inhale:* Lift into Bridge.

- *Exhale:* Lower back down to floor.

SUPPORTED BRIDGE

- Lift hips and place a yoga block or bolster beneath the hips, lower, and rest on the support.

DRAWBRIDGE

- Lift and lower each leg, one leg at a time, extending the leg straight up, without sagging the hips, as if to allow tall boats to pass.

> ### Caution!
>
> Gaze straight up when practicing Bridge; turning the head when the spine is lifted can strain the neck.

>> **See this pose in a lesson:** stress busting (page 167), energy equalizing (page 170), good posture and strong core (page 177), digestive support (page 188), teen restorative (page 211)

Reimagine the Pose!

Shield • Rainbow • Trapdoor • Humpback Whale

Famous Bridge (for example: Tower, Sydney Harbor, or Golden Gate bridges)

UPWARD FACING BOW

Urdhva Danurasana

What Is Upward Facing Bow and How Does It Help?

Upward Facing Bow is a strong back-bending pose and inversion. A full body posture, the whole body is stretched, making this pose super energizing.

 Simple Steps for Kids

* see page 114 for pose illustration

- Begin in Bridge (page 115).

- Place your hands on the yoga mat, framing your face, palms down and fingertips pointing to the shoulders.

- Lift your hips and straighten your arms, placing the crown *lightly* on the floor (support your weight with the hands and feet).

- *Inhale:* Use your hands and feet to push the floor away and lift your body into an arched shape. Straighten your arms and legs as much as you can.

- *Exhale:* Rest your head between your arms. Breathe slowly and fully while holding this shape.

- To exit, *inhale* and tuck your chin toward your chest. *Exhale:* Slowly and carefully lower your head, shoulders, and back along the floor a vertebrae at a time.

TIP: If you don't have the strength to lift and hold this pose safely, practice Bridge.

» See this pose in a lesson: energy equalizing (page 170), positive body image (page 191)

Reimagine the Pose!

Arch • Cave • Wheel • Ferris Wheel • Energy Circle

KNEES TO CHEST

Apanasana

What Is Knees to Chest and How Does It Help?

Practicing Knees to Chest garners the benefits of a forward bend while lying on your back! A restorative pose to counter backbends, Knees to Chest gently stretches the hips and lower back.

Simple Steps for Kids

- Begin by lying on your back.
- Hug both knees in toward your chest.
- Wrap your forearms around your legs, below the knees at the top of the shins.
- Relax the upper body on the floor.

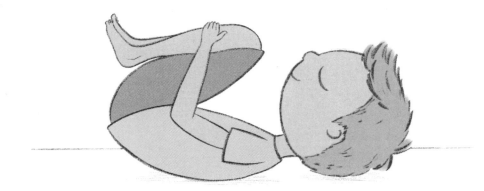

TIP:

- If wrapping the arms is too challenging (due to tight shoulders—perhaps from too much computer use), place the hands on the tops of the shins.

- ***Love your body:*** Hug your knees and legs and thank them for all of the hard work they do each day!

Variations

ROCK 'N' ROLL

- Hug knees to chest and gently roll back and forth along the spine. Practice this to provide tactile input to help calm and organize the nervous system, strengthen core muscles, and massage the back.

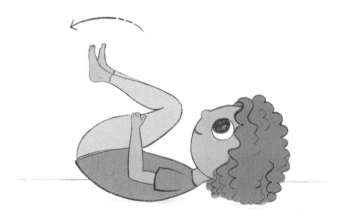

rock 'n' roll

>> See this pose in a lesson: chilling out (page 173), good posture and strong core (page 177), digestive support (page 188), positive body image (page 191), shape (page 196), teen restorative (page 211)

Reimagine the Pose!

Full Moon · Ball of String · Snail · Beach Ball · Sea Urchin

HAPPY BABY
Ananda Balasana

What Is Happy Baby and How Does It Help?
Happy Baby is a restorative, relaxing hip stretch and lower back release.

Simple Steps for Kids

- Lie on your back; hug both knees to your chest.
- Grip the outer edge of each foot with your hands and guide your knees toward your armpits.
- Flex your feet and relax your upper body on the yoga mat.
- Be still like a dead bug, or gently rock from side to side like a happy baby.

TIP: If you cannot reach your feet, hold onto the back of your thighs instead.

>> See this pose in a lesson: stress busting (page 167), digestive support (page 188), bee (page 199), teen restorative (page 211)

Reimagine the Pose!
Dead Bug ▪ *Baby Spider*
Bug on Its Back
Pig Rolling in Mud
Wrestler

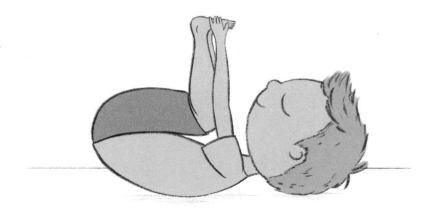

WIND RELIEVING POSE

Pavanmuktasana

What Is Wind Relieving Pose and How Does It Help?

Wind Relieving Pose is a gentle stretch and release for the hips and lower back. As its name suggests, this pose supports digestive health.

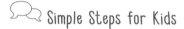 Simple Steps for Kids

- Lie on your back.

- Hug your right knee in toward your chest and clasp your hands at the top of the right shin. ***Inhale.***

- ***Exhale:*** Guide the knee toward the right armpit, thigh parallel with your torso.

- Hold and breathe. Release and repeat on the left side.

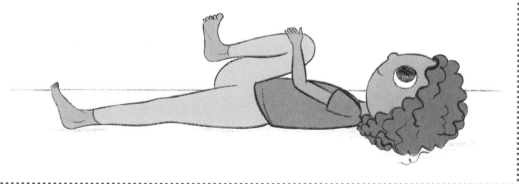

» **See this pose in a lesson:** good posture and strong core (page 177), digestive support (page 188), teen restorative (page 211)

Reimagine the Pose!

One-Legged Frog · Sprouting Seed · Runner · Sleeping Flamingo · Turkey Leg

WATERFALL

Viparita Karani

What Is Waterfall and How Does It Help?

Waterfall is a relaxing and restorative supported inversion.

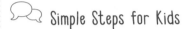 Simple Steps for Kids

- Begin in Supported Bridge Pose (page 116) with hips lifted and resting on a yoga block or bolster.
- Relax the arms alongside your torso, with the palms down.
- Lift both legs straight up in the air, feet and knees aligned with the hips, and flex your feet.
- Imagine your legs are a beautiful cascading waterfall.

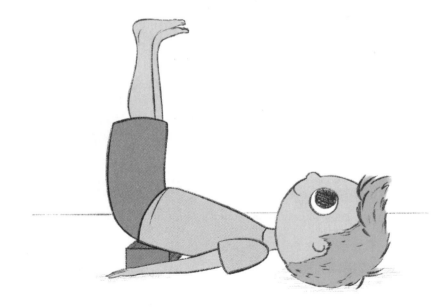

Variations

If your child has trouble straightening or holding his legs in this position, try the following variations.

LEGS UP THE WALL

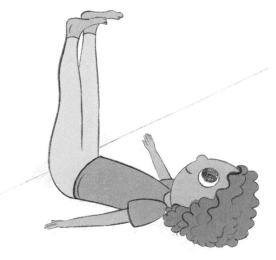

- Sit with one side of your body as close to a clean wall (i.e., no shelving, artwork, etc.) as you can.

- Roll onto your back and swing your legs up to rest against the wall.

- Your hips may have moved away from the wall; in this case, scoot your butt closer.

- Allow the legs to relax into the support of the wall as your upper body rests on the floor.

legs up the wall

LEGS ON A CHAIR

- If you don't have wall space, place a chair at one end of the yoga mat. Rest your calves on the seat of the chair as your torso relaxes on the floor.

>> See this pose in a lesson: chilling out (page 173), allergies and colds (page 184), partner (page 206), teen restorative (page 211)

Reimagine the Pose!

Fruit Bat · Exclamation Point · Ice-cream Cone · Rocket Ship · Cascading Falls

PLOW
Halasana

What Is Plow and How Does It Help?

Plow is a backbend, hip stretch, and inversion that helps develop balance and core stability.

 Simple Steps for Kids

- Lie on your back, arms alongside your torso, with your palms facing down.

- Press your arms into the floor and swing your legs behind your head.

- Tuck your toes and press back through the heels to lengthen and straighten your legs along the floor above your head. Align your hips with the shoulders.

- Bend your elbows and place your hands on your mid-back, fingers pointed straight up. Gently press your elbows into the floor and your hands into your back to support the spine.

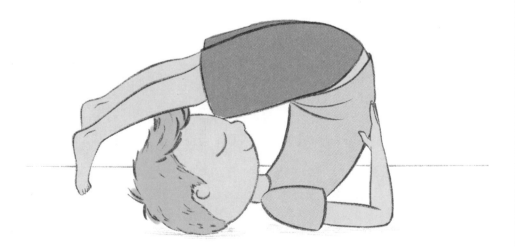

Modifications

If your child's legs do not make contact with the floor, cue her to bend her knees and frame her face with her legs.

Variations

BICYCLE PLOW

- Lift your feet away from the floor and bicycle the legs, maintaining Plow Pose.

TIP: If your child goes too fast when cued to bicycle the legs, ask her to pretend she is cycling up a really big hill. The resistance will make her pedal super slow.

>> **See this pose in a lesson:** energy equalizing (page 170), chilling out (page 173), good posture and strong core (page 177), digestive support (page 188), positive body image (page 191), beach adventure (page 202)

Reimagine the Pose!

Tipper Truck • Slippery Slug • Dancing Caterpillar • Sow the Soil • Paddleboat

SHOULDER STAND

Sarvangasana

What Is Shoulder Stand and How Does It Help?

Shoulder Stand is a balance challenge, inversion, and core-stabilizing pose. Turning the body upside down serves as a reminder that it's possible to view things from a different perspective.

 Simple Steps for Kids

- Lie on your back with your knees bent.
- Lift your legs away from the floor and toward your face until your hips and back also lift away from the mat.
- Bend at the elbows and place your hands on your back for support.
- Float your legs straight up overhead. Ideally, the shoulders, hips, and feet align in this pose. Walk your hands up your back, toward the mid and upper back areas, and press your elbows and upper arms into the floor for support.
- Gaze at your feet—*never turn your neck in this pose*. Flex your toes toward your face to keep your feet and legs engaged and strong.

TIP: If your child does not have the strength to support himself safely in Shoulder Stand, work on Bridge (page 115) first. Practice Drawbridge (page 116), lifting one leg at time, extending the leg straight up, without sagging the hips.

» **See this pose in a lesson:** energy equalizing (page 170), good posture and strong core (page 177), positive body image (page 191)

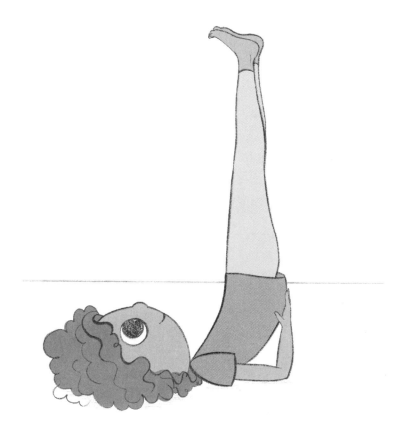

Variation

SHOULDER STAND BICYCLES

• Bicycle the legs while holding Shoulder Stand, moving only the legs; keep the upper body, torso, and core aligned and strong.

TIP: If your child goes too fast when cued to bicycle his legs, ask him to imagine he is bicycling in taffy or chewing gum and has to move really, really slow.

Reimagine the Pose!

Lollipop • Laser Beam • Bowling Pin • Candlestick • Sunflower

FISH

Matsyasana

What Is Fish and How Does It Help?

Fish is a backbend and inversion that expands the chest and shoulders and stretches the neck. Practicing Fish counters hunched and rounded shoulders from computer use, and it's a great pose to practice following Shoulder Stand (page 126) to gently stretch the shoulders after balancing on them.

 Simple Steps for Kids

- Lie on your back with your arms resting alongside your torso, palms down.
- Lift one hip at a time, placing each hand—palm down, fingers pointing to the feet—beneath each hip, so the hips rest on top of both hands.
- *Inhale:* Bend the elbows and lift and puff your chest. Create a shelf with the forearms to support your upper body.
- *Exhale:* Drop your head back and rest the crown *lightly* on the floor.
- Place *very little* weight on the crown of the head; it should barely touch the floor.

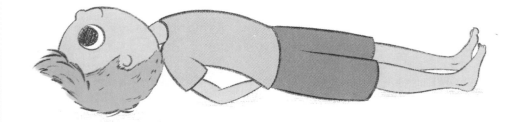

Variation

If your child is not strong enough to hold Fish or can't do Fish due to tight shoulders or a shoulder injury, try Supported Fish, a restorative variation that offers the same benefits.

SUPPORTED FISH

- Position a bolster horizontally on the yoga mat, toward one end.
- Lie on your back, aligning the shoulder blades over the bolster.
- Open and expand your arms to rest on the floor, palms facing up.

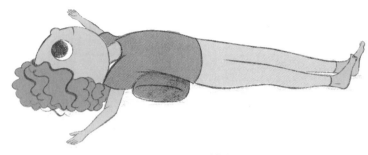

supported fish

TIP: If extending the neck is uncomfortable, support the head with a pillow.

>> **See this pose in a lesson:** energy equalizing (page 170), allergies and colds (page 184), positive body image (page 191), teen restorative (page 211)

Reimagine the Pose!

Backward Dive • Puffer Fish • Manatee • Stargazer • Rippling Water

DOUBLE KNEE RECLINED TWIST
Supta Matsyendrasana

What Is Double Knee Reclined Twist and How Does It Help?

Double Knee Reclined Twist is a pose that gently stretches the hips and lower back. Spinal rotation experienced in this pose improves and supports spine flexibility.

Simple Steps for Kids

- Lie on your back with the knees bent, feet flat on the floor.
- Extend your arms to rest on the floor in a T shape, at shoulder height, palms down. *Inhale.*
- *Exhale:* Lower both knees to the right.
- *Inhale:* Bring knees back to center.
- *Exhale:* Lower knees to the left.

Variations

WHALE BREATH

- Move your knees to the center on each inhale, and to the right or left with each exhale. Continue flowing from side to side, moving the legs in sync with your breath.

SUPPORTED RECLINED TWIST

- Place a bolster or pillow beneath the legs and small pillow between the knees. Hold and relax before switching sides.

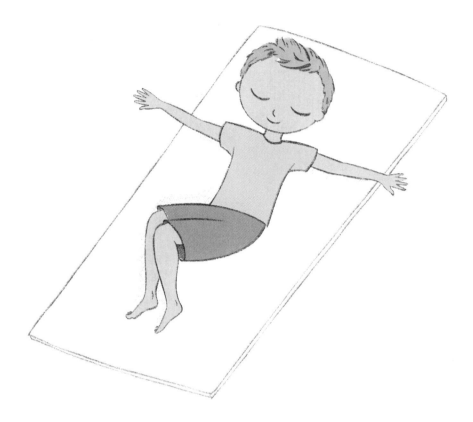

» **See this pose in a lesson:** chilling out (page 173), good posture and strong core (page 177), allergies and colds (page 184), digestive support (page 188), beach adventure (page 202), teen restorative (page 211)

Reimagine the Pose!

Comet's Tail • *Lightning Bolt* • *Swimming Whale* • *Windshield Wipers* • *Blowing Breeze*

FINAL RESTING POSE
Savasana

What Is Final Resting Pose and How Does It Help?

Typically cued at the end of a yoga session, Final Resting Pose provides the opportunity to rest and relax. This is an ideal pose to practice breathing, meditation, and guided relaxation, or simply to chill out.

Simple Steps for Kids

- Lie on your back.
- Rest the arms alongside your torso with the palms facing up, or fold your arms and place your hands on your belly.
- Separate the legs and allow your feet to flop open.
- Relax your entire body. Imagine sinking into the support of the floor or yoga mat beneath you.

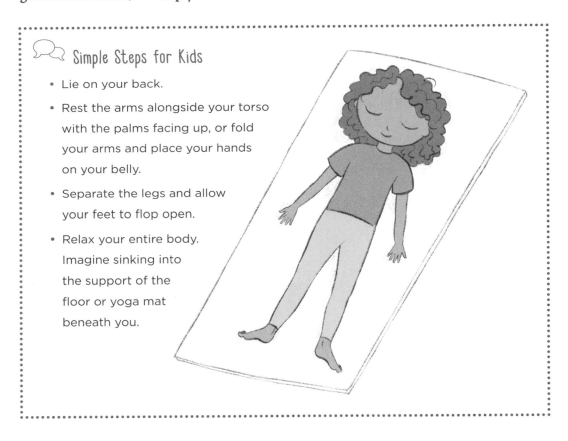

Reimagine the Pose!

Puddle • Melted Wax • The Big Relax • King of Calm • Floating Star (Snow Angel variation)

Variations

Help your child settle into Final Resting Pose by ironing out any remaining kinks in his body with these variations.

- **SNOW ANGEL:** *Inhale* and open arms and legs wide; *exhale* and draw legs together and arms alongside the body.

- **NO:** Gently roll the head from side to side, moving slowly with the breath.

- **WINDSHIELD WIPER FEET:** Gently rock the feet from side to side.

- **KNEE HUG TO CHEST:** Give yourself a *big* hug, breathe in, and breathe out to release the body into Final Resting Pose. Relax.

TIPS: Teach your child the importance of relaxation! Taking breaks to rest and restore will make her more productive at school and play. The following tips will enhance her relaxation experience:

- Place a pillow, bolster, or rolled blanket under the knees to support the lower back.

- Support your child's head with a soft pillow.

- Use an eye pillow.

- Play gentle, relaxing music.

- Use a blanket (swaddle your child like a burrito—young children love this). Make it cozy—warm the blanket in the dryer!

- Allow plenty of time for your child to enjoy Final Resting Pose.

Modifications

Young children may not stay still in this pose for long periods—a short story or yoga *nidra* relaxation for young children may be helpful (see page 176); tweens and teens will be happy to relax and restore for 15 to 30 minutes.

>> See this pose in a lesson: stress busting (page 167), chilling out (page 173), good posture and strong core (page 177), positive body image (page 191), shape (page 196), beach adventure (page 202), teen restorative (page 211)

CHAPTER FOUR

Essential Elements

Yoga is like a good peanut butter and jelly sandwich—the poses are the peanut butter, delicious but incomplete without sweet jelly and yummy bread to hold it together! This chapter includes vital ingredients—breathing, centering, warm-up, and relaxation techniques—to complete your child's yoga experience and help you to create a perfect yoga PB&J. Explore the suggested warm-ups, breathing, and relaxation techniques in this chapter, mix in your child's favorite yoga poses, and create an awesome yoga adventure to nurture your child's whole health and happiness.

Breathing and Centering

Breathing is a big part of yoga. Chapter Three (page 21) details how to cue your child through the incremental stages of fifty poses, using the breath as a tool to support alignment and safe stretching. Breathing and centering techniques are highly encouraged at the beginning of a yoga practice to center your child and clear her mind, preparing her to connect intentionally and mindfully with her body as she moves through her yoga practice. A yoga practice, without mindfulness, would be plain old stretching and, reflecting on my PB&J analogy, practicing yoga without breathing and centering is akin to making a PB&J without jelly and bread. Here are some fun ways to center and prepare for yoga, unless otherwise instructed, these can easily be accessed seated in Easy Pose (page 26) or standing in Mountain Pose (page 42).

CIRCLE-PASS

An ideal activity for busy, fidgety hands, Circle-Pass provides the opportunity to learn how to control the hands and body in a positive way.

What Do You Need?

All you need are two or three juggling scarves per child; you can make your own by cutting out small squares of silk or tulle—or simply use tissues.

Simple Steps for Kids

- Begin with two scarves.
- Toss one scarf in the air and, at the same time, pass the second scarf across to the hand that released the first scarf.
- Catch the first scarf in the hand that released the second scarf and, at the same time, release the second scarf into the air.
- Continue moving the scarves in a constant circular motion.
- Bring attention to your breath. Are you breathing or are you holding your breath?
- Focus on your breath and relaxing your body as you continue to move the scarves in a circular motion. Relax your shoulders, jaw, and face.
- If you can easily move two scarves in a circle for a long period, try adding a third.

TIP: Is your child having trouble with two scarves? Use one! Coordinating and maintaining a circular motion with even one scarf requires focus.

No Props? No Problem!

Use beanbags or rolled-up socks. Tennis balls are also a good idea, but I prefer softer items when working with children.

>> See this in a lesson: focus (page 163)

TWISTER BREATH

Twister Breath slows the breath to calm the nervous system and relieve stress and anxiety. This technique supports the development of concentration and motor planning skills.

 ## Simple Steps for Kids

- Sit in a comfortable seated position. Place the tip of your right index and middle fingers at the top of your nose, between the eyebrows, and gently press your right nostril closed using your thumb.

- *Inhale* through your left nostril, then lightly press that nostril closed with your ring and pinkie fingers.

- Release your thumb from your right nostril and *exhale* slowly and fully through that nostril.

- Keep the right nostril open and *inhale* fully before closing it off with the thumb.

- Release your left nostril and *exhale* slowly and fully out of the left nostril. This completes one cycle. Repeat for several cycles.

TIPS:

- If your child is left-handed, reverse this exercise.

- Cue young children, who have undeveloped fine motor skills, to use the index finger of each hand to close and release each nostril.

» See this in a lesson: focus (page 163), tech support (page 181), allergies and colds (page 184)

SOOTHING BREATH

Soothing Breath calms and soothes the body and mind. The placement of hands on the heart and belly provides tactile input to self-soothe, as well as physical feedback from the breath moving in and out of the body.

 ## Simple Steps for Kids

- Sit in Easy Pose (page 26) or rest on your back.
- Place one hand, palm down, over your heart and the other hand, palm down, on your belly. Relax your elbows and shoulders.
- Slow down your breath, feeling the chest and belly expand beneath your hands as you breathe in and relax as you breathe out.
- Relax and enjoy slow, controlled breaths. Notice the soothing and calming effect on your mind and body.

» See this in a lesson: stress busting (page 167), teen restorative (page 211)

SUN BREATH

Sun Breath is an energizing technique that is especially helpful to release tension in the jaw and mouth area.

 ## Simple Steps for Kids

- **Inhale** through your nose and reach your hands toward the sky; imagine grabbing the sun in both hands.

- Quickly pull your hands back toward you, palms flat and facing the middle of your torso. Open your mouth and **exhale,** making a "ha!" sound. Imagine pulling the energy and power of the sun into your core, or power center.

Variation

MOON BREATH:

Slowly reach both hands to the moon on a count of five—wiggle your fingers to grab the moon. Exhale super slowly to a count of five and lower your hands, gently placing the moon on your belly.

>> **See this in a lesson:** energy equalizing (page 170), chilling out (page 173)

SUNSHINE BREATH

Sunshine Breath is a centering technique that links gentle body movement to the breath cycle.

 ## Simple Steps for Kids

- *Inhale:* Sweep the arms up in a big circle until the palms meet high above your head.

- *Exhale:* Keep the palms pressed together and draw them down toward the middle of your chest or your heart.

- *Inhale:* Keep the palms pressed together and straighten the arms back up overhead.

- *Exhale:* Circle the arms back down alongside the torso. This is one complete round. Repeat several rounds.

TIP: Remind your child to link his body movement to his breath. Each movement should match his inhale and exhale. Like a car that does not move without gas, his body should not move without an in or out breath fueling it.

>> **See this in a lesson:** energy equalizing (page 170), bee (page 199), beach adventure (page 202), partner (page 206)

BELLY BREATHING

Belly Breathing is a deep-breathing technique to relax the mind and body, and to ease stress.

 Simple Steps for Kids

- Lie on your back on a yoga mat. Breathe in, consciously filling your lungs all the way. When the lungs expand to capacity, the belly will rise.
- As you breathe out, be sure to fully empty your lungs. Pull your belly button all the way in, as if it could touch your spine. (This won't really happen, but it is a good visual to help you fully expel all the air.)
- Repeat for several rounds, until you feel calm and relaxed.

TIP: Help your child with a visual cue: Place her hands, a beanbag, a book, or a toy (such as a rubber ducky) on her belly to help her observe the effects of deep Belly Breathing. Or try Belly Boat Float variation.

Variation

BELLY BOAT FLOAT:

Place a paper boat on your child's belly so he can observe the boat moving up and down as he breathes in and out. As the captain of that ship, he'll discover he has complete control of its movement via the breath. If your child folds his belly boat prior to practice, he'll experience the art of origami, which is touted to be meditative, calming, and relaxing. Folding paper to create the boat improves hand-eye coordination, fine motor skills, and encourages patience as your child carefully learns to follow step-by-step instructions. If you can't remember how to fold a paper boat, there are plenty of online tutorials.

›› See this in a lesson: chilling out (page 173), digestive support (page 188), beach adventure (page 202), partner (page 206), teen restorative (page 211)

ELEVATOR BREATHING

Focusing on both the spine and breath in this exercise encourages the improvement of general posture; it also slows the breath to support relaxation.

 ## Simple Steps for Kids

- Begin in a comfortable seated position, hands resting on top of your thighs, shoulders relaxed, and eyes closed.

- Visualize your spine running from your tailbone all the way to your skull and imagine it is an elevator shaft, with an elevator cab that travels up and down your spine.

- As you breathe in, feel the spine grow light and tall as the elevator rises to the top floor—your head.

- As you breathe out, feel the elevator travel back down the spine all the way to the basement—your tailbone.

- Continue with Elevator Breathing for several rounds.

» **See this in a lesson:** good posture and strong core (page 177)

BUMBLEBEE BREATH

Bumblebee Breath tickles the mouth and lips and fills the whole body with the vibration and energy of one's own breath.

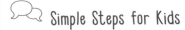

Simple Steps for Kids

- Cover your ears with your thumbs, blocking outside sounds. Gently wrap the remaining four fingers over your closed eyes.

- Take an easy breath in, filling up with air until the belly expands. *Exhale* through the nose with your lips closed, making a humming sound for the duration of your exhale.

- Repeat for several rounds.

» **See this in a lesson:** allergies and colds (page 184), bee (page 199)

Warming Up

Practiced independently, some yoga poses feel really good and are perfectly safe to practice cold. However, some can cause an injury if practiced without first warming and loosening the body to prepare it for deeper stretches. The following section features gentle to moderately paced warm-up sequences to help prepare your child's whole body for her yoga practice.

Eye Stretches

Often overlooked when stretching the body, the eyes have six muscles that control movement. While these muscles are not particularly strong, gentle eye stretches can help refresh tired and overworked eyes. Why would your child's eyes be overworked? Computers are typically the culprit—extended use, poor lighting, and the distance your child positions himself from the screen can all contribute to eyestrain.

RACCOON EYES

 Simple Steps for Kids

- Rub your palms together until your hands feel warm.

- Keep rubbing your hands as you breathe in.

- Gently place your warm palms over closed eyes as you breathe out.

- Hold your hands there, breathing normally. Relax and enjoy the warmth radiating from your hands until it naturally fades.

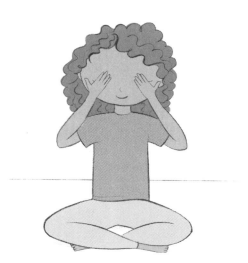

TIP: If your child wears glasses, remove them before practicing.

» **See this in a lesson:** tech support (page 181), allergies and colds (page 184)

ROLLY-POLLY-SUPER-SLOWLY

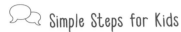 Simple Steps for Kids

- Sit comfortably and look straight ahead. Do not move your head at all during this exercise, simply move your eyes in each direction as far as you comfortably can, without straining.

STAGE ONE

- *Inhale:* Turn both eyes up, toward the ceiling. As you *exhale*, move both eyes to look right.
- *Inhale:* Lower your eyes down, toward your belly button. *Exhale:* Move your eyes to look left.
- Repeat three cycles in each direction.

TIP: Although moving in sync with the breath is not necessary for this eye stretch, I recommend it to inspire kids to move nice and slow.

STAGE TWO

- Look up with both eyes and *slowly* move eyes in a circle without stopping: up → right → down → left → up
- Repeat three times in each direction.
- Blink a few times and relax your eyes.

≫ See this in a lesson: tech support (page 181)

Tongue and Mouth Stretches

A muscular organ, the tongue has eight muscles that support its shape and position. Many breathing techniques stretch the tongue via tongue positioning. The following technique stretches the tongue and releases tension from the jaw and face.

LION'S BREATH

 Simple Steps for Kids

- *Inhale* deeply through your nose.

- Open your mouth wide, stick out your tongue, and *exhale* strongly while making a "ha" sound.

- Turn your eyes to look up toward the ceiling and stretch your hands and fingers to frame either side of your face like a lion's bushy mane.

- Repeat several times.

» **See this in a lesson:** stress busting (page 167)

Neck and Shoulder Stretches

Using computers, carrying heavy bags, poor posture habits, and sleeping in a strange position can all create tension and discomfort in the neck and shoulders. The following stretches loosen the neck and shoulders and relieve tension.

NECK AND SHOULDER STRETCH

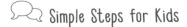 Simple Steps for Kids

- Rest the hands on your lap or thighs. Relax your shoulders away from the ears.

- *Inhale*, holding chin in a neutral position.

- *Exhale* and lower your chin toward your chest.

- Continue this for several rounds of breath, inhaling to lift chin to neutral and exhaling to lower it toward the chest.

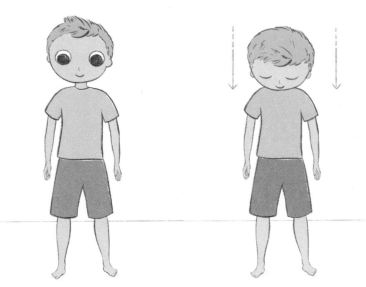

» **See this in a lesson:** tech support (page 181)

NECK ROLLS

 Simple Steps for Kids

- Rest the hands on your lap or thighs. Relax your shoulders away from the ears.

- *Inhale* with chin in neutral position.

- *Exhale:* Lower chin toward your chest.

- Be sure shoulders remain in relaxed position.

- Gently circle your chin toward the right shoulder as you inhale.

- *Exhale:* Move chin back to center, keeping it close to the chest.

- *Inhale:* Move chin toward your left shoulder.

- *Exhale:* Return to center.

- Continue rolling from shoulder to shoulder, connecting the movement to several rounds of breath.

- Upon completion of the final round, *inhale* to float your chin to a neutral position and *exhale* through an open mouth to help release any additional tension from the neck.

» **See this in a lesson:** chilling out (page 173), tech support (page 181)

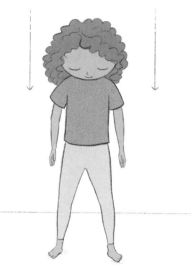

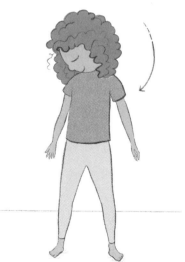

SHOULDER SHRUGS

💬 **Simple Steps for Kids**

- **_Inhale:_** Lift your shoulders up toward your ears.
- **_Exhale:_** Roll shoulders slightly back and down—imagine your shoulder blades sliding down your back.

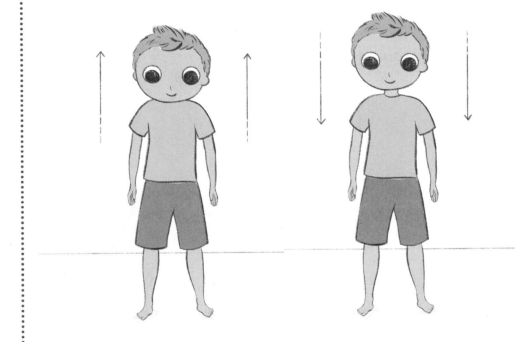

Variation

SWIMMING TURTLE:

Roll your shoulders backward and forward, or alternate shoulders like a swimming turtle.

» **See this in a lesson:** stress busting (page 167), chilling out (page 173), tech support (page 181)

Wrist and Hand Stretches

Hands can be busy. Nimble computer hands that industriously type away all day get tired and strained, as do swiftly swiping tablet hands and fingers, and our gaming friends' fast and furious console hands also need a break. Overuse is not the sole issue; the weight of gadgets, combined with your child's posture and hand positioning can strain wrists, hands, and fingers. Balance breaks from gadgets with the following wrist and hand stretches.

BACKWARD HANDS

 Simple Steps for Kids

- Extend the right arm forward, at shoulder height with the palm facing up.

- *Inhale:* Place your left hand on top of the right palm.

- *Exhale:* Gently bend the right wrist and fingers toward your body. Do not force the wrist backward; hold it at the point where you feel a *gentle* stretch in the wrist, and breathe slowly and steadily.

- Repeat on the left side.

» See this in a lesson: tech support (page 181)

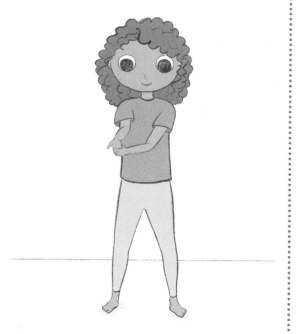

FINGER-TAPPING HAPPY BREATH

 Simple Steps for Kids

- *Inhale:* Spread the fingers and thumbs on both hands wide.
- *Exhale:* Tap the tip of your index finger to the tip of your thumb.
- *Inhale:* Stretch the fingers and thumbs on both hands wide.
- *Exhale:* Tap the tip of your middle finger to the tip of your thumb.
- *Inhale:* Open both hands wide, stretching the fingers and thumbs.
- *Exhale:* Tap the tip of your ring finger to the tip of your thumb.
- *Inhale:* Stretch the fingers and thumbs on both hands as wide as you can.
- *Exhale:* Tap the tip of your little finger to the tip of your thumb.
- Press both palms together, resting near your heart. Close your eyes, breathe normally, and think of something that makes you feel super happy.
- Repeat several times.

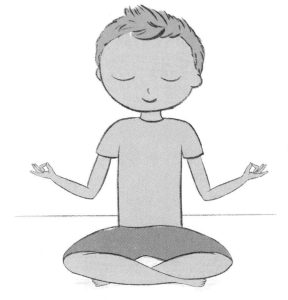

» **See this in a lesson:** tech support (page 181)

Full Body Warm-Ups and Stretches

Gentle, flowing body movements energize and warm up the body, preparing it for deep stretches and longer holds in yoga poses.

HIP CIRCLES

 Simple Steps for Kids

- Stand with feet hip-distance apart or wider, sit in Easy Pose (page 26), or sit in a chair with both feet on the floor.

- If you're standing, place your hands on the hips and begin to rotate the hips in a circular motion. Keep both feet grounded. If sitting, place hands on thighs or knees and keep both hips connected with the floor (or seat) and circle the upper body, moving from the hips.

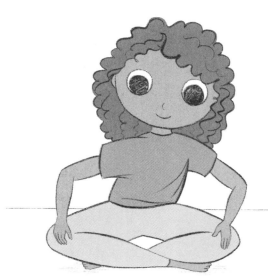

- Make the circles as big and slow as you like. Switch directions.

>> **See this in a lesson:**
shape (page 196), bee (page 199), teen restorative (page 211)

CAT-COW FLOW

 Simple Steps for Kids

- Cow: **Inhale**, dropping your belly toward the floor.
- Cat: **Exhale**, tucking in your chin and tailbone and arching your spine like a cat.
- Move back and forth between Cat and Cow poses, linking the body movement to your breath. See page 83.

» **See this in a lesson:** stress busting (page 167), good posture and strong core (page 177), tech support (page 181), digestive support (page 188), teen restorative (page 211)

CHILD'S POSE–DOG FLOW

 Simple Steps for Kids

- Begin in Child's Pose (page 111). Extend arms along the yoga mat in front of your body.
- **Inhale** to Table (page 81).
- **Exhale** to Downward Facing Dog (page 96).
- **Inhale** to Table.
- **Exhale** to Child's Pose.
- Repeat for several rounds.

» **See this in a lesson:** energy equalizing (page 170), good posture and strong core (page 177), teen restorative (page 211)

BASIC SUN SALUTATION

Energizing and centering, Sun Salutations modulate energy levels, warm up the body to prepare it for deeper stretches, and support a mind-body connection. Not all kids have trouble focusing, but many get a case of the sillies once in a while; a few rounds of Sun Salutation will work wonders to redirect that energy and prepare kids to focus or concentrate before homework, a test, lecture, or an important game.

Traditionally, several variations of Sun Salutation exist; below is a Basic Sun Salutation with suggested modifications to build upon, once your child warms up. Practice one or two full rounds of Basic Sun Salutation before introducing the build-on poses. Linking each movement to a breath is recommended, however: cue your child to use several breaths as she transitions from one pose to the next, or hold a pose if she needs to work on alignment or catch her breath.

 Simple Steps for Kids

- Begin in Mountain (page 42), standing at the top of your yoga mat.
- *Inhale:* Extended Mountain (page 43).
- *Exhale:* Standing Forward Fold (page 46).
- *Inhale:* Step left foot back to Low Lunge (page 53).
- *Exhale:* Step right leg back to Plank (page 88).
- *Inhale:* Hold Plank.
- *Exhale:* Lower to modified Low Push-Up with knees down (page 89).
- *Inhale:* Cobra (page 92).
- *Exhale:* Downward Facing Dog (page 96).
- *Inhale:* Step left foot forward to Low Lunge.
- *Exhale:* Step right foot forward to Standing Forward Fold.
- *Inhale:* Extended Mountain.
- *Exhale:* Mountain.

Modifications

Ready to build on the Basic Sun Salutation? Try these.

Substitute Extended Mountain with:

- Extended Mountain with Baby Backbend (page 43)

Substitute modified Low Push-Up with:

- Low Push-Up (body in one long line, don't drop knees; page 89)

Substitute Low Lunge with:

- High Lunge (page 53)
- Crescent Lunge (high or low with backbend) (page 52)
- Warrior I (page 50)

Substitute Cobra with:

- Upward Facing Dog (page 94)

➤➤ See this in a lesson: focus (page 163), energy equalizing (page 170), positive body image (page 191), beach adventure (page 202), teen restorative (page 211)

Core

Vital for supporting the back and trunk, the core (major and minor muscle groups within the trunk) supports the body's ability to balance, walk, run, and move! The following stretches strengthen and stabilize the core body muscles.

RACING CAR

 Simple Steps for Kids

- Lie on your back, with your arms resting alongside your torso, palms facing up.
- *Inhale:* Lift your shoulders and head off the floor and reach your hands toward your feet.
- *Exhale:* Flex your toes toward your face. Breathe steadily and hold.
- For additional core strengthening, gently rock from side to side and imagine steering a racing car around the track.

» **See this in a lesson:** good posture and strong core (page 177)

WATERWHEEL

 Simple Steps for Kids

- Lie on your back. Hug your knees to your chest and press your lower back to the floor.
- *Inhale:* Slide your hands to the tops of the knees and lower your feet toward the floor in front of the hips.
- *Exhale:* Hug the knees back into the chest.
- Repeat for several rounds.

» **See this in a lesson:** good posture and strong core (page 177)

SMALL BALL–TUG-OF-WAR

- Lie on back in Knees to Chest Pose (page 118).

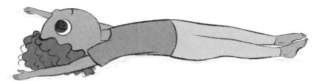

- *Inhale:* Extend your legs straight along the floor and reach your arms up past your ears. Stretch from your fingertips to your toes, like somebody has you in a tug-of-war.

- *Exhale:* Knees to chest, tuck your chin and make yourself into a small ball.

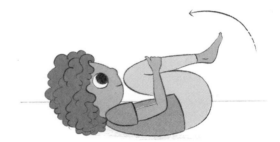

- Move with your breath—*inhale* to Tug-of-War, *exhale* to Small Ball—for several rounds.

›› See this in a lesson: good posture and strong core (page 177)

YOGA BICYCLES

 ## Simple Steps for Kids

- Lie on your back. Lace your fingers behind your head to support your head and neck.

- Lift your shoulders and head away from the floor, and keep your elbows wide.

- Lift your legs off the floor, bend your knees, and flex your feet.

- *Inhale* fully. As you *exhale*, extend your right leg out straight (hovering above the floor) and draw the left knee toward your chest. Guide your right elbow toward your left knee.

- *Inhale* back to center—head and shoulders lifted and gazing to ceiling, both knees bent and feet flexed.

- *Exhale:* Extend left leg out straight and draw right knee toward the chest. Reach left elbow toward the right knee.

- These are yoga bicycles! Continue riding your yoga bicycle for up to 1 minute, being mindful to keep your movements slow and controlled.

- For a bigger challenge, try bicycling the legs in Plow (page 124) and Shoulder Stand (page 126)!

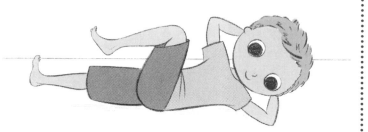

TIP: Bilateral coordination does not develop until 5 to 8 years of age. Support the upper body by propping it on bent elbows and slowly bicycle the legs.

>> **See this in a lesson:** digestive support (page 188), beach adventure (page 202)

Relaxation

Taking a little time at the end of practice to relax and restore is a key element that differentiates yoga from sports and exercise—I can think of no other physical activity that incorporates the concept of being completely still in order to absorb its physical and mental impact, before transitioning to other activities. Offering relaxation to your child at the end of her yoga practice teaches her to slow down and truly absorb life's experiences, instead of jumping mindlessly from one activity to the next.

There are many ways to offer relaxation to your child, from storytelling to guided imagery to listening to music. Expose your child to different experiences and see what she enjoys and finds most relaxing. This book includes one yoga *nidra* story (page 176) and two guided progressive relaxation scripts (pages 159 and 183) to help get you started. Yoga *nidra*, or yoga sleep, is a practice where the mind and body become deeply relaxed yet remain awake. Progressive relaxation is a method of mentally scanning the body, systematically relaxing one area at a time.

Storytelling captures the imagination and is a wonderful tool to engage young children in their relaxation experience. Snoozy-Doozy Naptime Yoga (page 174), features a yoga *nidra* story themed around the moon and stars. Close Down Your Apps and Recharge (page 183), a progressive relaxation technique adapted for shorter seated sessions, can be found at the end of Tech Support, a yoga sequence for desk and computer users (page 181). The following progressive relaxation technique, Your Amazing Body, fosters a positive body image for children.

YOUR AMAZING BODY

Focused on gratitude, the following progressive relaxation can be changed to anything your child may need—more love, energy, happiness, and so on. Simply substitute the gratitude language with words that support her needs.

- Gently close your eyes and settle against the support of your yoga mat and pillows.

- Let's take three breaths together.

- Easy *inhale* through the nose. Open mouth, *exhale*, relax your whole body. Repeat two more times.

- Breathe normally, without effort, allowing each breath to flow in and out of your body easily and gracefully, each breath ebbing and flowing like gentle ocean waves.

- As your breath moves in and out of your body, thank your body for this simple yet vital function. Say the words in your mind with each breath: as you breathe in, "thank," as you breathe out, "you."

- Send gratitude to your face, for its smiles and ability to communicate with others. Breathe in, "thank," breathe out, "you."

- Your amazing brain is a mini computer that works super hard. Breathe in, "thank," breathe out, "you."

- Curly, straight, short, or long, your hair makes you uniquely you. Breathe in, "thank," breathe out, "you."

- Your throat helps you to speak kind words and sing. Breathe in, "thank," breathe out, "you."

- Send gratitude to strong shoulders and arms. Breathe in, "thank," breathe out, "you."

- Say thank you to creative hands that write, play music, and bring life to your dreams. Breathe in, "thank," breathe out, "you."

- Feel your chest expand and relax accommodating each breath. Breathe in, "thank," breathe out, "you."

- Fill your belly with gratitude: It works hard processing food to keep you healthy and energized. Breathe in, "thank," breathe out, "you."

- Your strong back and core carry you every day. Breathe in, "thank," breathe out, "you."

- Thank your legs and feet: They allow you to walk, run, skip, and play. Breathe in, "thank," breathe out, "you."

- Thank your *whole* body. Breathe in, "thank," breathe out, "you."

- Your amazing body has so many parts that work in harmony to make you! Breathe in, "thank," breathe out, "you."

- Your amazing body keeps you healthy. Breathe in, "thank," breathe out, "you."

- Your amazing body makes you happy. Breathe in, "thank," breathe out, "you."

- Your amazing body can run, play, think, and create. Breathe in, "thank," breathe out, "you."

- Your body is a gift to love, cherish, and respect. Breathe in, "thank," breathe out, "you."

- Your amazing body is perfect in every way. Breathe in, "thank," breathe out, "you."

- Rest and relax—following each breath with gratitude, send your breath and gratitude anywhere in your body that needs a little extra love, or anywhere in your body you are especially grateful for. With each breath in, "thank," each breath out "you."

FIVE

Kids' Yoga Support

This chapter targets yoga practices to support common issues kids (and parents) experience, from the ability to focus to difficulty sleeping; it also includes a Healthy Kids section, offering yoga sequences to support children's health and wellness.

The poses and practices featured in each sequence can be found in Basic Posture Guide (page 21) and Essential Elements (page 134). Refer to these chapters for tips on safe cues, modifications, and alignment instruction. Each sequence features suggested cues to support your child as she holds and transitions to and from poses. If you find the pose names, themes, or cues are too juvenile for your child, switch it up; refer to the posture guide for alternate suggestions and the English and Sanskrit names for each pose, or make up your own. Yoga is flexible—the sequences in this book have been created to inspire you and your child to explore yoga in a fun and playful way, so get creative and have fun with your child.

> Yoga support is suggested strictly for symptomatic relief—a doctor must be consulted to treat and diagnose the cause of any conditions or symptoms your child may be experiencing. Your doctor or health-care provider should be consulted prior to practicing any of the sequences and practices suggested in this book.

Hocus Pocus, I Can Focus
Yoga for Concentration, Focus, and Self-Regulation

Yoga can be a wonderful tool for children to learn self-regulation skills; however, some children are challenged when it comes to quieting the mind and stilling the body. Many parents dismiss the notion of yoga, fearing their kids are too impulsive, too loud, too distracted, too . . . well, you name it, I've probably heard it! The following practice is designed to engage kids in focus-based activities that direct the mind to present moment-to-moment awareness via active play, accompanied with a selection of grounding and slightly to moderately challenging yoga poses. Grounding poses help to center kids energetically—think of flighty, unfocused behavior as the wind or air; to balance this energy, we need a strong foundation to feel anchored or grounded to the earth. Challenging poses require focus to practice them successfully and are a great way to center busy minds.

I themed the poses with a magic theme, but you can switch it up to appeal to your kids—sorcerers, wizards, witches, or warlocks are all interchangeable, according to your child's preference. For older kids, drop the theme altogether and cue poses in traditional Sanskrit or English. Complete the sequence as a whole, or cherry-pick practices that are most helpful for your child. Remind him he can access many of the techniques on his own, anytime he needs—if standing in Tree Pose for a few rounds of breath helps him to focus prior to a test at school, encourage him to do so.

HOCUS POCUS I CAN FOCUS YOGA

» Warm-Up

MAGICAL SUN DANCE: Sun Salutations (page 153). Practice two or three rounds of Basic Sun Salutation to warm up; if this is too challenging for your child, begin with the circle-pass activity below.

» Centering

JUGGLING: Circle-Pass (page 135). "Work your magic with some juggling fun!"

» Yoga Adventure

MARVELOUS MOUNTAIN: Mountain (page 42). "Look at this marvelous mountain, tall, still, and strong."

WIZARD WARRIOR: Warrior I (page 50)—right side first. "Touch your palms overhead to make a pointy wizard's hat. Hold still and breathe; imagine what spells you might cast."

CAST YOUR SPELL: Warrior II (page 55)—right side first. "Stretch your arms to cast your spell."

POUR MAGIC POTION: Triangle (page 57)—right side first! "Pour the magic potion to complete your spell."

MARVELOUS MOUNTAIN: Mountain. "Return to your marvelous mountain and imagine what spell your wizard will cast next."

Repeat Warrior I through Triangle on the left side.

MARVELOUS MOUNTAIN: Mountain. "Return to your marvelous mountain, tall, strong, and still."

MAGIC CAPE: Warrior III (page 62)—right side. "Put on your magic wizard's cape and prepare to fly!"

MOUNTAIN POSE: Mountain. "Land wherever you like. Stand still for a moment, taking it all in."

MAGIC CAPE: Warrior III—left side. "Put your magic cape back on and fly home."

FLYING WITCH: King of the Dancers (page 76)—right and left sides. "Past the flying witches to your right . . . and . . . the witches to your left."

ENCHANTED TREE: Tree Pose (page 73)—right and left sides. "Over enchanted woods, filled with magic trees."

MARVELOUS MOUNTAIN: Mountain. "Return to your marvelous mountain, tall, strong, and still."

MAGIC SORCERER'S STAFF: Staff Pose (page 30). "Be still and strong, like a magic sorcerer's staff."

BALANCING ACT: Boat (page 34). "Master a balancing magic trick."

TRANSITION: Roll forward to Table (page 81) and Plank (page 88).

SORCERER'S SWORD: Plank. "Find your sorcerer's sword."

MAGICAL MYSTICAL FLOATING TRICK: Side Plank (page 89)—right and left sides. "Use your sorcerer's skills to master a magical, mystical, floating trick!"

TIP: Add Tree legs (page 90) for an extra challenge or drop your bottom knee if Side Plank is too challenging.

» Closing

TRICKY BREATH: Twister Breath (page 136). "Muster up those sorcerer skills to practice tricky breath!"

» Modifications for Kids

Challenge your child further with these modifications:

MAGICAL MINDFUL CHALLENGE FOR KIDS

Complete the following postures from the above sequence by balancing a small bean-bag on your head: Mountain, Warrior I, Warrior II, King of the Dancers, Tree Pose, Staff Pose, Boat. Increase the challenge by transitioning from one pose to the next without dropping the beanbag.

HEALTHY COMPETITION

How long can you hold the pose? Aim to hold the pose a little longer each time you practice—competing only with yourself, of course! Using a timer is a great idea, but counting your breath is even better, as it will keep your mind focused while holding the pose.

» Tips for Parents

MAGIC MANTRA

Because mantras are personal, I encourage students to find a mantra that resonates with them. However, the following mantra (which happens to be my own personal mantra) is one I happily share with my students: "Where is my body? Where is my breath? Where is my mind?" This simple cue effectively reminds children to check in with the three things they *can* control: their body, their breath, and their mind. It truly works like magic, uniting the body, breath, and mind with the present moment. Use this mantra as a cue throughout class, and encourage kids to adopt it throughout their day, not just while practicing yoga.

PRAISE AND REWARD

Be sure to reward your child by pointing out successes—kids who struggle with impulsive behavior and the inability to focus are often picked on all day long for what is perceived as negative behavior. It is empowering for children to learn that, with a little practice, they *can* be successful at focusing their minds and regulating their bodies, even if it is just for a moment. If you reward that success, your child will want to build on it.

Stress Busters
Yoga for Stress and Anxiety Relief

Stress and anxiety are not exclusively adult issues; in fact, many children struggle with stress and anxiety. It may be episodic, triggered by peer pressure, death, divorce, illness, pressure at school or overscheduling; or it may be clinical—a medically diagnosed stress or anxiety disorder.

Yoga can be very beneficial for children struggling with stress and anxiety—breathing and meditation techniques typical to yoga are helpful tools to regulate stress and self-soothe, and, physically speaking, a good yoga stretch can iron out kinks in the body caused by stress-related tension. Your child will learn about her body and identify where she tends to carry tension. Common areas include the jaw, shoulders, stomach, and fists. Knowledge is power: If your child understands her habits, she can begin to access breathing and stretching techniques before tension, stress, and anxiety escalate.

The following sequence includes challenging and grounding poses as well as practices to slow and regulate the breath. Challenging poses require your child's full attention to practice, distracting her from pesky, anxious thoughts and diverting her mind from stress triggers. They also teach her to breathe and find a sense of calm, even when facing something difficult. Grounding poses provide a sense of stability and safety. Learning to breathe fully, slowly, and deeply, your child will gain the tools to shift herself from fight-or-flight-activated stress-breathing patterns to a calm, controlled response.

The sequence can be completed as shown, or you can jump to the portion most helpful for your child in the moment. I call this sequence King of Calm, but it is adaptable for queens, too. The most important lesson to teach your child is that she reigns over her kingdom and can master her response to stressful situations.

KING OF CALM YOGA

» Centering

KING OF MY BREATH: Soothing Breath (page 137). Begin in Easy Pose (page 26) and place one hand on your heart and one hand on your belly. Feel your breath expand into both hands as you inhale, and sense your whole body relax as you exhale. Connect a mantra to each inhale and exhale.

> ### Suggested Mantras
>
> Is your child having trouble coming up with a mantra that inspires? Here are some suggestions (replace "KING" with "QUEEN," where it is relevant):
>
> - *Breathe In* **I AM KING**, *Breathe Out* **I AM CALM**
> - *Breathe In* **KING OF MY BODY**, *Breathe Out* **KING OF MY HEART**
> - *Breathe In* **I AM STRONG**, *Breathe Out* **I AM CALM**
> - *Breathe In* **KING OF MY MIND**, *Breathe Out* **KING OF ME**
> - *Breath In* **KING OF THE JUNGLE**, *Breathe Out* **KING OF THE BIRDS**
> - *Breath In* **I RULE MY KINGDOM**, *Breathe Out* **I AM THE KING OF CALM**

» Warm-Up

KING OF THE JUNGLE: Lion's Breath (page 145). "I'm king of the jungle! I'm king of how I feel. Hear me roooaaar! I let go of stress and tension!"

CARE-FREE LION: Shoulder Shrugs (page 148). "Who cares? Who cares? No worries, no cares. I'm a care-free lion; I'm not hiding away in a turtle shell!"

BRAVE, FEARLESS LION: Lion's Breath. "I'm a brave and fearless lion! Hear me yell!"

BIG CAT: Cat-Cow (page 83). "No worries can break me, my back is strong and can carry the load. I bend and flex and go with the flow."

TRANSITION: Tuck toes, lift knees from floor, and pounce forward to the top of the yoga mat.

» Yoga Adventure

SILLY CAT: Standing Forward Fold (page 46). "Pouncing forward I dance the sillies and stress away, bowing to another king."

THE KING OF PRIMATES: Gorilla (page 48). "King of the primates, my muscles are strong and my fur unruffled."

TRANSITION: Release grip from under feet and slowly roll upper body to standing position. "Even when I am feeling small, there's a gorilla inside me standing tall!"

THRONE: Chair (page 68). "I'm king of calm, sitting in my throne."

ROYAL STRENGTH: Balancing Chair (page 69). "I draw strength from my crown all the way to my toes."

HUMBLE SUPPORT: Twisting Chair (page 69)—right and left sides. "Even kings ask for help; I look around and draw strength from my friends."

KING OF THE BIRDS: Eagle (page 71)—right and left sides. "I'm king of the birds. My keen vision sees clearly, and my wings help me soar."

TRANSITION: Table through to Child's Pose.

SOLID ROCK: Child's Pose (page 111). "I'm solid as a rock—cool, still, and strong."

TRANSITION to lie on your belly.

REGAL SPHINX: Sphinx (page 95). "I'm regal as the mystical sphinx basking in the sun."

TRANSITION to lie on your back.

KING'S MOAT: Bridge (page 115). "Wise kings build moats to connect castles, kingdoms, and communities."

FALLEN KING: Happy Baby (page 120). Roll the wrists and ankles, and gently rock on your back. "We all fall down or face struggles, like a bug on his back. But we can help ourselves, by being king of calm or asking others for help."

KING OF CALM: Final Resting Pose (page 132). Rest and relax, or reconnect with the Soothing Breath and mantra you started class with.

TIP: A small bag of rice placed on your child's belly and an eye pillow will provide additional sensory input to calm and relax the nervous system.

·············· Energizer Equalizers: ··············
Yoga to Regulate Energy Levels

The energy-equalizing practices in this chapter do double duty—working well to refresh sluggish and lethargic kids while effectively harnessing and redirecting their excess energy when they become super excitable.

Vinyasa flow (linking body movement to breath) yoga works for both ends of the energy spectrum. Moving the body in time with the breath provides a controlled outlet for excess energy, bringing a sense of order and control to the body and mind. Dynamic movement linked to the rhythmic flow of the breath helps to get the blood pumping to wake up tired, sluggish bodies and minds. The Sun Salutations cued in this sequence are slightly more challenging than the Basic Sun Salutation outlined in the Essential Elements chapter (page 134). In this sequence you are encouraged to include invigorating backbends and balance challenges such as Crescent and Lunge poses (page 52) instead of Warriors to help ignite energy in tired kids, and anchor excess energy in overly excited children.

Be mindful of your goals when offering this sequence to your kids: backbends are invigorating and energizing, so if you notice arousal levels increasing, redirect that energy by cueing forward bends. The postures have been marked for your convenience—BB for backbends and FB for forward bends—allowing you to adapt this sequence to benefit your child's energy levels.

THE ENERGY IN *ME* YOGA

» Centering

Choose the technique that bests suits your goal.

Finding energy—I'm feeling sluggish and need to perk up! SUN BREATH (page 138). "Bring the sun's energy to you so you can get out and play."

Redirecting energy—I'm feeling silly; let's harness that energy! SUNSHINE BREATH. "Paint the sun on the sky."

» Warm-Up

DANCE FOR THE SUN: Sun Salutation (page 153). Warm up with three to five full rounds of Sun Salutation. See sidebar below for tips to make it more challenging.

Build on Sun Salutations!

- **MOVE FROM COBRA (PAGE 92) TO UP DOG (PAGE 94):** Be a snake basking in the sun's warmth or a strong wave responding to the moon's magnetic pull.

- **SUBSTITUTE LOW LUNGE (PAGE 53) WITH HIGH LUNGE (PAGE 53):** Balance the energy between your feet to be stable and strong.

- **LOW OR HIGH LUNGE WITH LATERAL BEND:** Be the sun chasing the moon away.

- **LOW OR HIGH LUNGE WITH BACKBEND:** Reach back and feel the sun's energy fill your heart.

» Yoga Adventure

POWER OF WIND: Locust BB (page 104). "The power of the wind enables planes and birds to fly."

ENERGY CIRCLE: Bow BB (page 106). "Energy flows in a circle . . .

PUPPY CHASING HIS TAIL: Child's Pose–Dog Flow FB (page 152). ". . . like a puppy chasing his tail."

THIRSTY CAMEL: Camel BB (page 108). "Energy helps thirsty camels find water . . .

BURROWING BUNNY: Rabbit FB (page 110). " . . . and a bunny to burrow his home."

BRIDGE: Bridge BB (page 115). "Energy is water flowing under the bridge . . .

CAVE: Upward Facing Bow BB (page 117). ". . . into a cave."

DANCING CATERPILLAR: Plow (page 124). "It is the dancing caterpillars performing . . .

TALL SUNFLOWER: Shoulder Stand (page 126). ". . . beneath the tallest of sunflowers . . .

FISH: Fish BB (page 128). ". . . and fishes swimming in a pond."

SANDWICH FOR FUEL: Seated Forward Fold FB (page 32). "You have all of this in you but you still need fuel! Let's make a yummy sandwich . . .

Practice three rounds of Seated Forward Fold, holding on the third round:

1. "Butter your bread!"—your legs are the bottom piece of bread.

2. "Fill your sandwich with something yummy!"—lettuce, tomato, or ham.

3. "Relax and refuel"—the upper body is the top slice of bread. Hold Seated Forward Fold and breathe as you refuel.

ROLLERBLADES: Head to Knee Pose FB (page 36)—right and left sides. ". . . before a skate in the park."

Practice three rounds of Head to Knee Pose on each leg, holding the forward fold on the third round:

1. "Pull your skate onto your foot."

2. "Lace up your skate boot."

3. "Gracefully glide"—hold and breathe, imagine skating gracefully.

» Closing

ENERGY IN *ME:* Easy Pose (page 26). Seated meditation: select a breathing technique to meet your goal—remember, your needs may have shifted during this class.

SUN BREATH: "Bring the sun's energy to you so you can get out and play."

SUNSHINE BREATH: "Paint the sun on the sky."

· · · · · · · · · · · · The Chill Zone · · · · · · · · · · · ·
Yoga for Relaxation and a Better Night's Sleep

Sleep (or the ability to deeply relax) can be an elusive dream for many, including children. Winding down and disconnecting from a busy day with a simple yoga routine can prepare the body and mind for a better night's sleep (or a daytime nap). Many of the yoga poses in the following Snoozy-Doozy Naptime Yoga routine are grounding and supportive—sending the message to the brain and body via the nervous system that it is safe to let go, slow down, and relax. Some of the yoga poses selected for this routine apply gentle pressure to the body, either through positioning, movement, or the use of props, providing sensory input to modulate arousal levels and help kids calm down and chill out.

The following routine can be practiced in its entirety, or choose one or two poses to practice with your kids before bed, either on a yoga mat close to the bed, a place where your child naps, or on the bed itself. Practice each pose for at least three to five full rounds of breath.

SNOOZY-DOOZY NAPTIME YOGA

» Centering

MOON ROCK: Supported Child's Pose (page 113). Left cheek down, face right with eyes closed. Inhale: "Feel your back expand as it fills with breath, you are a giant moon rock." Open mouth—exhale: "Imagine magic moon dust filling the room."
Switch—right cheek down, face left with eyes closed, and repeat.

TIP: Parents gently rub your child's back as they hold moon rock—the tactile input will encourage relaxation and direct your child's awareness to the back part of his body where you are guiding him to expand with each breath.

TRANSITION slowly from Child's Pose to Easy Pose (page 26).

MOON BREATH: Variation of Sun Breath (page 138).

» Yoga Adventure

HALF-MOON CIRCLES: Neck Rolls (page 147). "Look down at the moon you placed on your belly and draw half-moon circles with your chin."

Repeat three to five rounds and slowly lift the chin back to neutral position after completing final round.

SHINING STAR SHOULDER SHRUGS: Shoulder Shrugs (page 148). "Feel your heart expand and shine, like a bright shining star."

TRANSITION slowly to lie on the yoga mat or bed.

ROCKET SHIP: Waterfall (page 122). "Raise legs straight up in the air like a rocket ship shooting into space."

TIP: For extra support, practice Legs Up the Wall variation (page 123). If near a wall—roll to one side and relax for a few breaths before slowly moving away from the wall and back to bed or the yoga mat to transition to the next pose.

STILL MOON: Knees to Chest (page 118). "Imagine you are a perfectly still round moon."

ROCKING MOON: Rock 'n' Roll (page 119). Rock side to side, and back and forth.

Tip: If your child has not yet developed the core strength required to roll side to side, or back and forth, assist him by placing one hand at the base of his neck and one on the back of his thighs and help him move gently and slowly.

STILL MOON: Knees to Chest. "Perfectly round, perfectly still!"

SHINING STAR: Reclined Bound Angle (page 29). "Stretch arms out and imagine you are a bright, shining star resting in the sky."

ROLLING MOON: Rock 'n' Roll. Rock side to side, and back and forth.

COMET'S TAIL: Double Knee Reclined Twist (page 130)—right and left sides.

FLOATING STAR: Snow Angel (page 133). "Imagine you are a star floating in space."

ROCKING MOON: Rock 'n' Roll. Rock side to side, and back and forth.

STILL MOON: Knees to Chest. "Curl up into a small moon."

» Relaxation

PUDDLE OF MOONLIGHT: Final Resting Pose (page 132). "Relax and melt your body, feel it spread out, like a puddle of moonlight."

TIP: Place a pillow under your child's knees and head for support, and cover him with a cozy blanket to be sure he is super supported and warm.

GLOWING MOON BELLY BREATH: Belly Breathing (page 140). Relax your hands on your lower belly and relax your shoulders and elbows. Feel your belly expand like a bright glowing moon with each inhale, and allow it to fade and relax as the belly softens with each exhale.

» Tip for Parents

Be sure that your child is tucked in and comfortable; you may want to snuggle with your child for the relaxation portion of this practice. Share a favorite story or offer guided relaxation. A simple, guided relaxation story for kids, on page 176, ties into the moon and stars theme from this practice. Feel free to get creative and come up with a story of your own.

Guided Relaxation/Yoga Nidra Story

"Imagine you are the brightest star, floating in space. A bold, shining light that can be seen from every corner of the world! Float freely, weightless in space, knowing that you are safe and supported, no matter how deeply you relax. Wiggle your toes, feel them twinkle and shine, then let them relax. Wiggle your fingers, feel them sparkle and glow, then let them relax. Wiggle your nose, feel it glimmer and glitter, and then relax. Each time you breathe in, imagine a bright light filling your star, making it shine, and each time you breathe out, the light softly fades as the skies switch from night to day and your star takes a well-deserved nap. Float and relax in the sky, supported, and relaxed. Each time you breathe in, your star glows bright; each time you breathe out, relax your star a little bit more as it fades and rests, waiting for night to return. Easy inhales, bright light filling your entire body—like a glowing, shining star. Relaxing exhales, fading, softening, resting . . . deeper and deeper with each breath out."

» Relaxation Tips

Enhance your child's relaxation experience with a heated blanket, extra pillows, or eye pillows—if he responds well to these props and likes them, be sure to include them each time you practice! Heated blankets do not have to be electric—warm a blanket in the dryer prior to your bed- or naptime yoga routine, and it will cool down naturally as your child drifts off to sleep.

Offer instructions to your child in a soothing whisper and gently assist her during this practice—these tactile and auditory cues encourage deep relaxation.

Instrumental music or nature sounds foster relaxation—I use gentle piano music, or instrumentals such as "Brahms's Lullaby." There are plenty of free or low-cost apps featuring multiple sound effects or music, from gentle night rain to falling stars. Find what your child responds to and use that.

Healthy Kids
Yoga Tips for Health and Wellness

Yoga can be a supportive practice for symptomatic relief, but it is not suitable for diagnosing or treating medical conditions; only your doctor or medical professional can do that. Please check with your doctor prior to practicing yoga with your child and always be aware of how your child is feeling—energy levels, presence of fever, and so on. Sometimes rest truly is the best medicine.

If you've practiced yoga with your child before, guide him to reflect on how he feels and what type of yoga practice he thinks would be most helpful. Does he need to focus on breathing? Would guided relaxation be beneficial? Does he want to get up and move or opt for a gentle, slow stretch? A strong element of yoga is cultivating self-awareness and wisdom to understand our own bodies and minds, and nurture them with practices that are beneficial.

As with all practices in this book, the following are mere suggestions; you are free to choose alternate poses and practices from the Basic Posture Guide (page 21) and Essential Elements (page 134).

Yoga Support for Good Posture and a Strong Core
Whether you are a child or an adult, poor posture can lead to tension, pain, headaches, insomnia, and low self-esteem; poor posture negatively impacts vital bodily functions such as breathing and digestion. In growing children, correct posture supports structural, neurological, and psychological development, and is vital to optimal health and wellness. Yoga can be instrumental in teaching kids how to develop and maintain good postural habits that will, quite literally, carry them through life.

The following practice includes stretches to warm up, lengthen, bend, flex, and rotate the spine, improving general flexibility and spinal health. Core-strengthening exercises are included to develop a strong core and support the spine and trunk.

So many children are hunched forward from using computers and tablets that I've dedicated an entire practice to focus on the neck, shoulders, wrists, and eyes (see Yoga Support for Tech Users, page 181). These practices are very supportive for healthy spines and encourage good posture. I highly recommend you teach both to your children, encouraging body awareness and empowering kids to correct poor posture habits and create healthy ones, especially when using computers.

STRONG, LONG, AND FLEXIBLE YOGA

Let's explore things that are strong, long, and flexible—just like you!

›› Centering

WORLD'S TALLEST BUILDING ELEVATOR: Elevator Breathing (page 141). Begin in Easy Pose (page 26) or Mountain Pose (page 42). "Imagine you are the world's tallest building. Your breath drives the elevator up and down, so people can journey to the top floor and enjoy seeing the world through your eyes."

›› Warm-Up

MOVE WITH THE WIND: Even the tallest buildings are designed to be flexible, so they can move with the wind. Imagine your breath is the wind, as you move through the following two flows, maintaining length in your spine and a strong core to support your tall skyscraper:

- Cat-Cow Flow (page 152)—repeat five times.
- Child's Pose–Dog Flow (page 152)—repeat five times.

›› Yoga Adventure

TRANSITION to Table (page 81).

- *SNAKES—Snakes have super long spines with as many as 200 to 400 vertebrae!*

SNAKE HIDING IN CAVE: Thread the Needle (page 86). "A snake's flexible spine allows him to curl, slither, and glide into caves and crevices." Switch sides!

HISSING SNAKE: Cobra (page 92). Inhale to lift into Cobra Pose, hold, and exhale with a long "hisss." Inhale to lift and lengthen your Cobra, and exhale to lower. Repeat three times.

STRIKING SNAKE: Upward Facing Dog (page 94). Only your feet and hands touch the floor, feel your long snake body lengthen from the tail (toes) to the hood (head). Hold striking snake for one full round of breath, and lower with your exhale. Repeat three times.

FLYING SNAKE: Locust (page 104). Snakes can't really fly, but they lift their tails and upper body to strike and swing. Keep your snake's belly down, and lift your hood and tail from the ground. Repeat three times, lifting your body a little bit higher each time. Lift and hold on the final round for up to three full breaths.

FLEXING SNAKE: Bow (page 106).

SLEEPING SNAKE: Child's Pose (page 111). Rest your busy hissing, striking, flying snake.

- **DOLPHINS**—*Dolphins have strong, flexible spines and tails to power them through the water when they swim and play.*

DOLPHIN SWIMMING: Dolphin Pose (page 98). Yogi's choice! Hold Dolphin Pose or swim like a dolphin. Here's how: Begin in Dolphin Pose, inhale, and lean forward so your head and shoulders come past your elbows. Exhale and press back to Dolphin Pose. Move back and forth with your breath.

GLIDING DOLPHIN: Dolphin Plank (page 91). Hold Dolphin Plank and imagine you're a dolphin gliding through the water. Don't forget to breathe. Dolphins never hold their breath!

DOLPHIN TAIL: Crocodile (page 103). Rest your head on your palms, bend your knees, and swish your strong dolphin's tail from side to side.

TRANSITION: Lie on your back.

- **BRIDGES**—*Strong and robust bridges are designed by architects to connect land and allow cars and people to safely travel over water, cliffs, ravines, and busy roads.*

BRIDGE: Bridge (page 115). Build a strong bridge.

DRIVE A CAR OVER BRIDGE: Racing Car (page 155). Cars pass safely over strong bridges.

DRAWBRIDGE: Drawbridge (page 116) or Rolling Bridge (page 116). Drawbridges open and close, allowing tall boats to safely pass.

PADDLEBOAT FLOATING UNDER BRIDGE: Waterwheel (page 155).

- **ROPE**—*A length of rope can be short or long, but to do its job and support and tether heavy items, it must be strong!*

UNBREAKABLY STRONG: Small Ball–Tug-of-War (page 156). Rope used in tug-of-war games is unbreakably strong!

- **TALLEST SUNFLOWER**—*With a little nurturing and patience, the tiniest seed can transform into the tallest, brightest sunflower.*

SEED: Knees to Chest (page 118). Curl into a small ball and imagine you are a seed soaking up all of the earth's nutrients, ready to sprout and grow into the tallest, brightest sunflower!

SOW THE SOIL: Plow (page 124). Prepare the soil to plant sunflowers!

GATHER SEEDS: Rock 'n' Roll (page 119). Gather sunflower seeds.

TRANSITION to Table (page 81) or Downward Facing Dog (page 96).

PLANT SEEDS: Half Pigeon (page 100). Plant the seed (placement of front leg) and cover it with soil (upper body resting over front leg). Switch sides!

TRANSITION: Lie on your back.

SPROUTING SEED: Wind Relieving Pose (page 121). Stretch one leg out along the floor to grow roots. Gently bend and draw the other knee close, as your seed sprouts and presses through the earth. Switch sides!

SUNFLOWER: Shoulder Stand (page 126). Stretch your toes to the sky, like a beautiful, tall sunflower!

TRANSITION: Slowly lower your body and lie on your back.

- **WHALES**—*Just like a dolphin, the whale has a strong, long, and flexible spine to help him navigate the deepest of oceans.*

SWIMMING WHALE: Whale Breath (page 130).

SLEEPING WHALE: Double Knee Reclined Twist (page 130). Hold and breathe. Rest your whale's tail to one side—imagine your whale taking a nap. Switch sides.

» Relaxation

FLOATING WHALE: Final Resting Pose (page 132). Prop a pillow, rolled yoga mat, or bolster under your knees to support your whale's tail. Imagine floating through the ocean, like a big powerful strong whale.

Yoga Support for Tech Users

Teaching kids body awareness and yoga exercises to counter computer and tablet use, and support the eyes, wrists, neck, and shoulders is vital—computers and tablets are not going away. The best we can do is educate our children how to safely use these tools and keep themselves healthy while doing so. The following sequence can be completed in its entirety, while sitting at a desk, or individual stretches and practices can be selected and used as mini breaks to stretch and refocus your child's mind and keep her body safe while using a computer or tablet. I recommend my students take a 30- to 60-second computer break every 20 to 30 minutes, selecting one stretch from the sequence to practice each time. I've gone with a high-tech theme here, but if your child is not into that, it's okay; simply use the original names (also provided) or offer the stretches by body part—eye stretches, neck and shoulder stretches, and so on.

» Centering

OPTICAL ORBS: Raccoon Eyes (page 143). Warm your hands like lasers and rest your palms over your closed eyes. Relax and enjoy the warmth of laser hands charging your optical orbs.

OCULAR BINOCULAR: Rolly-Polly–Super-Slowly (page 144). Fine-tune eye muscles with super-slow control. Be sure to move in both directions!

SOFTWARE PROGRAM CHECK: Twister Breath (page 136). Make sure your software (breath) is running well and smooth; you will need to access your software throughout the remainder of this tech-support tune-up.

» Yoga Adventure

CRITICAL HARDWARE MAINTENANCE: Backward Hands (page 149).

DIGITAL DIGIT TUNE-UP: Finger-Tapping Happy Breath (page 150).

ACTIVATE CYBORG CONNECTOR: Neck and Shoulder Stretch (page 146).

HI-TECH NECK: Neck Rolls (page 147). Access your internal software (breath) to gently swivel your high-tech neck from side to side.

AUTOMATION ROTATION: Shoulder Shrugs (page 148).

SOFT-WIRED LIMBS: Eagle (page 71). Follow cues for the arms only.

DRONE DROID: Take flight—sit squarely on a chair, both hips connecting with the seat and feet grounded on the floor in front of you. Reach your arms behind you, thumbs down and palms facing in, grip the sides of the back of the chair toward the bottom (if this is unavailable, grip the outer edge of the seat where it meets the back of the chair). Inhale to lengthen spine; exhale . . . gently lean forward, expanding the chest and stretching your arms and shoulders—hold and breathe.

HI-TECH FLEX: Seated Lateral Bend (page 45).
TIP: Make this a wrist and finger stretch, too: Interlace fingers and flip palms to face out; lengthen the arms away from your body at chest height. Inhale and reach arms overhead, lengthening from

hips to palms. Exhale. . . . Soften the shoulders away from the ears. Move through several rounds of Seated Lateral Bend in each direction.

MECHANICAL MOVEMENT: Seated Cat-Cow (page 84).

PROGRAM ROTATION: Seated Slide Twist (page 40).

BIONIC STRETCH: Seated Dog (page 97).

DEACTIVATE: Seated Forward Fold (page 32) in chair. Move the chair away from the desk or turn your chair 90 degrees to allow space for your body. Imagine your body is a robot deactivating. Gently fold your upper body over your legs and rest.

» Relaxation

Close Down Your Apps and Recharge

- Sit upright in your chair and close your eyes.

- Gently press your feet and hips into the floor and seat, so you are supported, upright, and aligned. Relax your shoulders down your back; soften your face and rest your hands on your lap or thighs.

- Imagine you are a tablet or smartphone. You've been working hard, almost all your apps are open and running, and your battery is beginning to fade. You need to close down your apps so you can recharge and feel refreshed. Let's journey through your apps, closing each one down for a much-needed rest.

- *The head app:*

  › The brain. Imagine your brain resting inside your skull. Gently close it down and allow it to relax.

  › The mind. A sub-app of the brain. Allow the mind to relax. It may try to turn itself back on, but remember, you're the boss! Allow the mind app to fade away. You can do it. Fade the apps for your brain and mind, to recharge and rest.

- *The face app:* "This is a very busy app—close it down and allow it to rest."
  - › Allow each of the face's sub-apps to relax as they close down: the temples, forehead, eyebrows, eyelids, eyelashes, and eyeballs. The nose, cheeks, ears, jaw, mouth, teeth, and tongue.
- *The neck and shoulder apps:*
  - › Relax your throat, neck, and shoulders as each app closes down for a well-deserved rest.
- *The arm apps:*
  - › Feel your arms, hands, and fingers relax as you close down the app for each arm, restoring the arms, hands, and fingers.
- *The torso app:*
  - › Allow the chest, belly, and spine to relax—closing down each torso app.
- *The leg app:*
  - › Switch off the app for the legs, ankles, feet, and toes. Both legs and feet completely surrender.
- All your apps are closed, your whole body is resting and recharging . . . deeply relaxed.
- Imagine being refueled with vital energy. Draw that energy up through your feet, and feel it soar throughout your entire body. What color is that energy? Imagine it filling every part of your body, revitalizing it.
- Sit quietly, resting and recharging for as long as you need.

Yoga Support for Seasonal Allergies and Colds

While a regular yoga practice can help improve overall health and boost immunity, it's fair to say that even the healthiest of kids will succumb to a cold at some point, and many healthy children can be affected by seasonal allergies. If your child has been exposed to a cold virus or suffers from allergies, yoga can't change that, but it may be helpful in supporting symptomatic relief.

The following sequence includes postures and practices that gently compress and massage sinus pressure points to relieve discomfort from built-up fluids and inflammation. Gentle inversions and forward folds may seem counterintuitive; however, after reverting to an upright position, excess fluids often drain away. Common cold medicines and steroids, used to treat allergies, can negatively impact digestion (causing constipation or diarrhea), so twists are included in the sequence to support healthy digestion—a key component of optimal immune function.

Experiencing a cold or allergies can leave one feeling tired, cruddy, and cranky. This slow-paced practice is designed to be supportive, nurturing, and restorative . . . just like a cup of warm chicken noodle soup.

TIP: Don't forget to keep tissues on hand, this practice may stimulate and relieve blocked sinuses, causing little noses to run!

EASY-BREEZY, I'M BREATHING EASY YOGA

» Centering

I DESERVE IT FACIAL MASSAGE:

- Use your middle and index fingers to gently press around the eye sockets. Be careful not to touch your eyes or eyelids; just gently press your fingers into the bony parts around your eyes. It may feel tender, like you are touching a bruise. Mucous and fluids build up in our sinuses (located at the center of the forehead, between the eyes, behind the nose, and on the cheeks) when we have colds and allergies, and this gentle massage can help relieve some of the pressure created by this.

- Gently massage your temples in a slow circular motion; the temples are located on either side of your face between the tail of your eyebrows and hairline.

- Use your middle, index, and ring fingers to gently press across your forehead. Begin resting those three fingers, of both hands, in the center of your forehead, above your nose. Gently press and release, moving each hand away from the other, across the forehead toward the temples.
- Gently massage the temples in a slow circular motion.

MELTING MUCOUS: Raccoon Eyes (page 143). Relax and imagine the warmth of your hands melting that pesky mucous away.

BUZZIN' BREEZE: Bumblebee Breath (page 142). Buzzing bees create a buzzing breeze.

>> Yoga Adventure

FIRE-BREATHING DRAGON:

- **BUILD YOUR DRAGON'S LAIR:** Child's Pose (page 111). Gently roll your forehead from side to side to massage it, and get ready to wake your dragon up. Find stillness.
- **DRAGON BREATH:** Take an easy breath in. As you breathe out, open your mouth wide and sigh like a fire-breathing dragon.

ROLLING CROCODILE: Crocodile (page 103). Rest your crocodile's head on your crocodile hands and gently roll your head from side to side, giving yourself a crocodile-style massage. Bend your knees and swish your crocodile tail from side to side. Lower your legs and find stillness, letting your crocodile rest.

SLEEPY PUPPY: Downward Facing Dog (page 96) or Puppy Pose (page 97). Resting puppies don't pant, they breathe easy. Hold Down Dog or Puppy Pose, breathing smooth and steady like a sleeping puppy.

RAGDOLL: Standing Forward Fold (page 46). Be relaxed, floppy, and happy like a giant ragdoll.

FRESH MOUNTAIN AIR: Mountain (page 42) with Twister Breath (page 136) or Bumblebee Breath (page 142) if nose is blocked. Practice for up to five rounds to help clear sinuses.

FALLING LEAVES: Seated Wide Leg Forward Fold (page 60). Imagine a gentle wind blowing leaves to the ground. Gently float into this fold and use props to support your upper body as needed. Rest and relax like a fallen leaf.

BLOWING LEAVES: Revolved Head to Knee (page 37). Rotate and float gracefully like a leaf blowing in the gentlest of winds. Switch sides.

GIANT NOSE: Head to Knee (page 36). Make a giant nose with your legs and breathe easy. Switch sides.

PUFFER FISH: Supported Fish (page 129). Puff your chest like a giant puffer fish and forget the wheeze—you're creating more space in your chest to breathe.

RELAXING BUTTERFLY: Reclined Bound Angle (page 29). Support your relaxing butterfly with a pillow or bolster propped under your back and head; this creates a mild and supported inversion to reduce postnasal drain that may tickle the throat and make your butterfly cough in a fully reclined position.

FLOWING BREEZE: Supported Reclined Twist (page 130).

» Relaxation

WATERFALL: Legs Up the Wall (page 123) or Legs on a Chair (page 123). Use an eye pillow—the weight of the eye pillow applies gentle pressure to help relieve sinuses and sends the message to the brain via the tactile system that it's time to relax. Prop head with a pillow if postnasal drip is causing a tickle or cough. Relax here as long as you can, breath flowing like a gentle, easy-breezy breeze.

Yoga for Digestive Support

Everybody eats and everybody poops, but, like many things in life, digestion does not always function smoothly. Digestive health effects overall wellness—from energy levels to immune function to mental and psychological health. Conversely, psychological issues, such as anxiety, can manifest as "tummy troubles" in children and adults alike. Eating a balanced diet, drinking plenty of water, and moving the body through play or exercise is extremely important when it comes to our digestive health, and, of course yoga can be very supportive in maintaining healthy digestion and resolving "tummy troubles."

The following yoga sequence, Tummy Yoga, supports healthy digestion—the routine encourages movement and is conducive to healthy digestion. The selected practices intentionally position the body to apply gentle pressure and massage the digestive track in the direction in which the system naturally functions—from ascending to transverse to descending colon. This supports healthy elimination and can help resolve common issues such as constipation and gas.

TUMMY YOGA

» Centering

HAPPY TUMMY BREATHING: Belly Breathing (page 140). Place your hands on your lower belly, fingertips touching in the middle to form a smile shape with your hands. Practice Belly Breathing for at least 2 minutes or longer, if possible.

Tips:

- Older kids should be able to practice this breathing technique for up to 5 minutes!

- Keep young children engaged by talking to them as they breathe and relax. Ask your child what she thinks would make her tummy smile. Encourage her to imagine she is filling her belly with those things each time she breathes in.

» Warm-Up

TRANSITION: Hug Knees to Chest (page 118) and gently Rock 'n' Roll (page 119) along your spine, arriving in a seated position. Move to Table (page 81).

SAGGING BRIDGE AND BIG BRIDGE: Cat-Cow Flow (page 152). Move slowly between sagging bridge and big bridge for three to five full rounds of breath.

DANCING LION (page 85). Be sure to move the hips from right to left, as this stimulates the digestive system from right to left. Balance out with a few counterclockwise circles, too.

» Yoga Adventure

BUTTERFLY/BAT: Bound Angle (page 27).

FLYING BUTTERFLY/BAT (page 28). Imagine your breath is the wind moving your butterfly/bat wings as you fly high up in the sky! Slowly rock knees up and down, linking each movement to your breath.

SNOOZING BUTTERFLY/BAT (page 28). Imagine your butterfly/bat taking a well-deserved snooze.

TRANSITION to Easy Pose (page 26).

BANANA BEND: Seated Lateral Bend (page 45). Stretch to the right side first—compressing and massaging the ascending colon. Stretch to the left side.

PRETZEL: Seated Twist (page 38). Twist to the right side first. Unwind and repeat on the left side.

TRANSITION: Lie on your back.

BICYCLE RIDE: Yoga Bicycles (page 157). Imagine peddling a bike through chewing gum or up a really, really steep hill! Move slowly and mindfully with each breath.

» Modifications

Bilateral coordination does not develop until 5 to 8 years of age—if this is too challenging for your child, cue him to prop up his upper body on his elbows and slowly bicycle his legs.

TRANSITION: Rock 'n' Roll (page 119) along the spine up to five times before arriving in a seated position.

FROG ON A LILY PAD: Squat (page 78). Sit still like a frog on a lily pad that is patiently waiting to catch a fly!

TRANSITION: Lie on your back.

PADDLEBOAT: Plow (page 124).

PADDLEBOAT CRUISE: Bicycle Plow (page 125).

If this is too challenging, hold Plow, or roll out of Plow and repeat Bicycle Ride.

PADDLEBOAT DOCK: It's time to dock your paddleboat! Place your arms alongside the torso for support and slowly roll out of Plow and lie on your back.

ONE-LEGGED FROG:

- Wind Relieving Pose (page 121) right side.
- Happy Baby (single leg, page 120) right side.

Repeat on the left side.

WHALE TAIL: Double Knee Reclined Twist (page 130) right side.

WHALE TAIL: Knees to Chest (page 118). Admire your beautiful tail!

WHALE TAIL: Double Knee Reclined Twist (page 130) left side.

Repeat the three stages of whale tail for several rounds, moving right to center to left.

TIP: This is my go-to practice when working with constipated kids. Slowly and mindfully swishing and admiring a gorgeous whale or mermaid tail is relatively restorative for kids who may feel icky and stuck from being constipated, and who lack the energy or desire to move a lot.

» Relaxation

BELLY BOAT FLOAT (page 140). Rest and relax.

» Teaching Tips

Modify the practice according to any gastrointestinal issues or symptoms that may be present. Always be sensitive to abdominal pain and how each movement or practice you offer effects your child; be prepared to modify the practice with supportive props such as pillows and bolsters, as needed. Move gently, incrementally building on how far your child moves into a pose, especially twists.

» Modifications

Encourage older kids and teens to take control of their health—talk to them about how the digestive system works and why it is important to maintain digestive health. Kids like to learn about their bodies, and by understanding something as simple as the direction waste moves in the body, they can access the poses on their own, if they experience discomfort at school or away at camp or a sleepover. Always encourage deep, slow, controlled breaths—this not only helps the body physically enter yoga poses without resistance but helps the mind to relax, too, relieving mental anxiety that often contributes to pesky tummy troubles.

Yoga to Support a Positive Body Image

Teaching kids to love, respect, and appreciate their bodies is vital to physical and psychological well-being. I am always surprised by just how early kids begin to make comments about being "skinny" or "fat"—judging and comparing themselves to others—even me! I have had girls as young as 8 years old ask if they will be as skinny as me if they practice yoga. Without skipping a beat I respond, "Forget skinny; you'll be *strong* and *healthy* if you practice yoga!" Sadly, I've had young children—boys and girls—tell me they are "too fat" to practice yoga, to which I respond, "You are beautiful [handsome] and absolutely perfect for yoga!"

My goal is to encourage kids to understand that while their bodies might look or function differently than others, yoga can help them build strength, flexibility, grace, self-respect, and self-love. Our bodies are amazing biological machines, a true source of awe and wonder. The following practice is designed to get kids connected to their body and explore how it can bend, balance, flex, and move in so many different and awe-inspiring ways.

I highly recommend encouraging your child with positive language such as "Strong Tree," "Fabulous Bow," and "Marvelous Wheel." Direct kids to fully explore each pose, noticing how it makes them feel, both physically and mentally. Perhaps your child feels confident after mastering Tree Pose, or has a profound sense of accomplishment when he balances in Half-Moon for the first time. How about that buzzing feeling he gets following a dynamic flow, when every cell in his body feels like it is vibrating? Direct your child's awareness to all the positive things he feels when practicing yoga and remind him that he created those sensations and feelings! It was his amazing body that moved in a way that made him feel relaxed, happy, stretched, vibrant, confident, and more. Such awareness develops appreciation, respect, and love for all the body does to support a healthy body image and strong self-esteem for your child.

MY *AMAZING* BODY YOGA

» Centering

MOUNTAIN WITH HANDS AT HEART (page 43). "Close your eyes and notice your breath. Slow down each inhale and exhale, connecting a mantra of your choosing to each breath."

Suggested Mantras

Having trouble coming up with a mantra? Here are some suggestions:

- *Breathing in,* I AM STRONG . . . *breathing out,* I AM HAPPY.
- *Breathing in,* I AM BRIGHT . . . *breathing out,* I AM HEALTHY.
- *Breathing in,* I AM BEAUTIFUL/HANDSOME . . . *breathing out,* I AM SMART.
- *Breathing in,* MY BODY IS STRONG . . . *breathing out,* MY BODY IS FLEXIBLE.
- I BREATHE IN AND SUPPORT MY BODY . . . I BREATHE OUT AND MY BODY SUPPORTS ME.
- *Breathing in,* MY MIND IS STRONG . . . *breathing out,* MY HEART IS HAPPY.
- I BREATHE IN AND LOVE MY BODY . . . I BREATHE OUT, MY BODY LOVES ME.
- *Breathing in,* I AM CONFIDENT . . . *breathing out,* I AM JOYFUL.
- *Breathing in,* I AM LOVED . . . *breathing out,* I AM FREE.
- *Breathing in,* I KNOW I AM ENOUGH . . . *breathing out,* I AM BRIGHT.
- *Breathing in,* I AM SAFE . . . *breathing out,* I AM HAPPY TO BE ME.

» Warm-Up

SUN DANCE: Sun Salutations (page 153). "Dance for the sun. Move your dynamic body and dance to the rhythm of your breath."

TIP: Build on Basic Sun Salutations to include Lunges, Warriors I and II, Upward Facing Dog, and Low Push-Up poses, as you feel ready. Practice at least five full rounds to really warm up your body!

» Yoga Adventure

STRETCHING DOG: Downward Facing Dog (page 96). "Enjoy the energy you created buzzing throughout your body as you lengthen and strengthen from your fingertips to your tail!"

GROUNDED WARRIOR: Warrior I (page 50)—right side. "Grounded and strong, my feet support me. Thank you, feet!"

GRACEFUL WARRIOR: Warrior II (page 55)—right side. "In quiet stillness, I find grace and strength."

STABLE AND STRONG: Triangle (page 57)—right side. "Stable and strong, my body supports me."

BRIGHT SHINING MOON: Half-Moon (page 66)—right side. "I glow like the moon and can balance, too!"

CONFIDENT KING/QUEEN: Chair (page 68)—"I'm confident as a king/queen perched upon his/her throne."

Repeat grounded warrior through bright shining moon on the left side. Return to confident king/queen once complete.

VITAL-I-TREE: Tree Pose (page 73)—right and left sides. "My body is vital and healthy, like a green leafy tree."

BEAUTIFUL BODY BOAT: Boat (page 34).

TRANSITION: Hug knees, tuck chin, and Rock 'n' Roll (page 119) along the spine, gaining momentum to roll through Table (page 81), and then lying on your belly.

FLYING FREE: Locust (page 104).

BOUNTIFUL BOW: Bow (page 106). "Like a strong bow, my body bends and never breaks."

TRANSITION: Lie on your back.

ENERGY CIRCLE: Upward Facing Bow (page 117). "A dynamic circle of energy, I'm radiant!"

PLENTIFUL PLOW: Plow (page 124). "Rolling into Plow with ease and grace, I appreciate everything I have and all I can do."

POISED SOLIDER: Shoulder Stand (page 126). "A tall, poised soldier, I stand proud and thankful. Proud of who I am, grateful for what I have."

BIG OPEN HEART: Fish (page 128). "With an open heart, I share my gifts with the world."

BIGGEST HUG: Knees to Chest (page 118). "I love my body; I'm so grateful for all it can do. There may be things that it can't master yet, and that's okay, too."

» Relaxation

THE *BIG* RELAX: Final Resting Pose (page 132). Repeat a mantra from one of the suggested mantras (page 168), or ask a parent or friend to read the progressive relaxation, Your Amazing Body (page 159), as you rest and relax.

CHAPTER SIX

Fun Themed Lesson Plans

The following chapter includes five complete lesson plans, one for each stage of child development—from toddler to young adult. Each plan includes suggested props and music so you can jump right in and begin sharing full-length classes with your child. Gender-neutral and age-appropriate, the plans can easily be adapted for children outside the specified age range; refer to Chapter Two (page 7) and adapt the plans by selecting practices to align with your child's developmental abilities.

SHAPE YOGA
Toddlers (18–36 months)

Shape yoga supports visual, verbal, and kinesthetic learning for your child to help her learn her shapes and colors while having fun. Your child may just be beginning to recognize shapes and colors at this age. Don't worry if she does not know all of them; you are here to help her! Practice time for this age is about 15 minutes.

TIP: You may want to introduce the concepts and theme of this lesson by reminding your toddler of the following: "Shapes are everywhere; they help us organize and identify objects. We can make shapes with our bodies, too, so let's play yoga and have fun creating shapes."

Suggested Props

- Colorful images of shapes
- Silk scarves

TIP: Support your child's ability to identify colors—use colorful silk scarves and images of shapes. Name the color and the shape each time you use the prop. For example "green triangle," "purple square," etc. Make your own reusable flash cards! Print images of shapes on index cards and laminate them.

Music

Add fun songs about learning shapes (such as "The Shapes Song" by Dream English or "Shapes Song" by The Kiboomers)—sing and dance along with your child to warm up. If lyrics are a distraction for your child, try instrumental music or no music at all.

Centering

BE THE WIND: Hold a scarf in front of your child's face and ask her to pretend she is the wind and blow on the scarf.

MAKE SHAPES:

- Spread the scarf on the floor in front of your child and make a square.
- Fold the scarf in half to make a rectangle.
- Unfold and turn the scarf 90 degrees to make a diamond.
- Fold the scarf in half to make a triangle!

RELAX: Help your child gather up the scarf into a tight ball, and hold it high over his head. Breathe in and then breathe out with a big sigh, letting go of the scarf. Encourage your child to feel as floppy as the scarf as it floats down.

TIP: Repetition supports learning at this stage, I recommend selecting three or four shapes per session. Introduce new shapes when you feel your child is ready.

Yoga Adventure

CIRCLE:

- Balloon Breath—Breathe in and sweep your arms overhead to make a balloon shape, exhale and lower them back down.
- Hip Circles (page 151). Imagine a colorful crayon sitting on top of your head and draw circles.
- Knees to Chest (page 118)
- Rock 'n' Roll (page 119)

DIAMOND:

- Bound Angle (page 27). Move your feet away from your body to make a diamond shape.

TRIANGLE:

- Seated Wide Leg Forward Fold (page 60). Sit with legs wide, this is a perfect triangle, or fold forward into a sleeping triangle.
- Triangle (page 57). This can be a tricky pose for this age—support and assist your child!

STAR:

- Fingers—Stretch your fingers into stars.
- Wide Leg Forward Fold prep pose (page 59). Make a star shape with arms and legs—do not fold forward. Stretch and wiggle your fingers to twinkle like stars.

CRESCENT:

- Standing Crescent Pose (page 44) or Seated Lateral Bend (page 45)

SQUARE:

- Table (page 81)

RECTANGLE:

- Reverse Table (page 82)
- Final Resting Pose (page 132). Rest arms alongside the torso and flex the feet to make the perfect rectangle shape.

Relaxation

CHILD'S POSE (page 111): Gently rub your child's back. Draw shapes on your child's back.

FINAL RESTING POSE: Gently massage your child's hands and feet and sing to her as she relaxes.

BEE YOGA

Preschoolers (3–4 years)

Bees may be known for stinging—*ouch*—but they also make yummy honey for us to eat. Bees need gardens full of beautiful flowers so they can make honey. In this yoga class, we will plant a garden on a sunny day, make some rain to help our seeds grow, and create blooming flowers to attract bees. Once our bees arrive they'll get busy making honey so we can create a sweet sandwich to eat. Yum!

Centering

LET'S MAKE A GARDEN TO ATTRACT OUR BEE FRIENDS!

- SUNSHINE: Sunshine Breath (page 139)
- PLANT SEEDS: Child's Pose (page 111)
- RAIN TO WATER SEEDS: Parents massage child's back with finger taps.

Yoga Adventure

OUR GORGEOUS GARDEN IS READY TO GROW!

- GROW TREES: Head to Knee Pose (page 36) but do not fold forward: Hold the leg position and reach your arms overhead like tree branches. Switch legs to grow an extra tree!

- BLOOMING FLOWERS: Press fingertips of both hands together to make a flower bud. Hold fingertips to nose and breathe in, smelling your beautiful flower. Gently open your fingers and blow on your blooming flower, spreading pollen to attract the bees.

HERE THEY COME—DO YOU HEAR THEM?

- BUZZING BEES: Bumblebee Breath (page 142)

- FLY LIKE A BEE: Bend elbows, place hands on shoulders, and circle arms backward and forward.

BE A GIANT QUEEN BEE!

- FLYING QUEEN BEE: Bound Angle (page 27). Flap your wings and fly!

- STRETCH ONE WING: Stretching Butterfly (page 28) with right leg extended

- HIDE IN YOUR HIVE: Snoozing Butterfly (page 28)

- FLYING QUEEN BEE: Bound Angle

- STRETCH YOUR OTHER WING: Stretching Butterfly with left leg extended

- HIDE IN YOUR HIVE: Snoozing Butterfly

- FLYING QUEEN BEE: Bound Angle

- STRETCH BOTH WINGS: Stretching Butterfly—both legs!

- HIDE IN YOUR HIVE: Snoozing Butterfly

- Repeat "Be a giant queen bee!" two more times!

DO BEES SNORE? NO, BUT MAYBE THEY BUZZ IN THEIR SLEEP . . . LET'S BUZZ, BEES!

- **BUZZING/SNOOZING BEE:** Snoozing Butterfly with Bumblebee Breath

BEES HAVE STINGERS!

- **RAISE STINGER:** Table (page 81). Lift your right leg in the air and point your toes. Imagine this is your stinger!
- **HIDE IN YOUR HIVE:** Child's Pose (page 111)
- **RAISE STINGER:** Table with left leg lifted
- **HIDE IN YOUR HIVE:** Child's Pose
- Repeat "Bees have stingers!" two more times.

DO BEES BUZZ INSIDE THE HIVE? WHO KNOWS?
LET'S HIDE IN OUR HIVE AND BUZZ!

- **BUZZ IN THE HIVE:** Child's Pose with Bumblebee Breath

BEES MAKE HONEY!

- **HONEY POT:** Triangle (page 57). Pour the honey from the honey pot! Be sure to pour from both sides of the honey pot!
- **STIR HONEY POT:** Standing Hip Circles (page 151)
- **TRANSITION** to Staff Pose (page 30) on the yoga mat.
- **HONEY SANDWICH:** Seated Forward Fold (page 32). Breathe in and reach up to grab the honey pot. Exhale, reaching for your toes, and roll back to seated Staff Pose, spreading the honey on your legs (the bottom piece of bread) with your hands. Repeat three more times: The third time, hold the forward fold, breathe, and imagine enjoying your yummy honey sandwich.

UH-OH! WE SPILLED SOME HONEY!

- **STICKY HONEY:** Seated Hip Circles (page 151). Move slowly—you're stuck in honey!

- **WIPE HONEY OFF:** Happy Baby (page 120). Rub hands and feet together and rock side to side to get that sticky honey off!
- **WIPE HONEY OFF:** Rock 'n' Roll (page 119). Get the sticky honey off your whole body!

UH-OH! WE ATE ALL THE HONEY!

Let's make a really big flower to produce lots of pollen and help our bee friends make more yummy honey.

- Human Mandala (page 234)

TIP: Just you and your child? No problem! You can make a flower mandala: Sit facing each other in Easy Pose (page 26), connect palm to palm with your child, raise up your hands as you breathe in, and lower them as you breathe out. Continue opening and closing your flower.

BEACH ADVENTURE YOGA
School-Age Kids (5–8 years)

This beach adventure class will have your kids playing on the beach, swimming, surfing, snorkeling, and relaxing. It doesn't matter if it is summer or winter, or if you live far away from the coast; with a little imagination, you can escape to the beach and enjoy a sunny yoga adventure.

Suggested Props
- Paper straws (bendy straws are best as they look like a snorkel)

Music
Ocean sounds, coupled with fun beach songs

Centering

SUNNY DAY: Sunshine Breath (page 139). The sun is shining. Where should we go?

BIKE TO THE BEACH: Yoga Bicycles (page 157). Jump on your bike; let's head to the beach!

SIT ON YOUR TOWEL: Easy Pose (page 26). Sit on beach towel (your yoga mat!) and trace the shape of your towel. This is your space on the beach (and in this class).

APPLY SUNSCREEN: Seated Forward Fold (page 32). Reach for your sunscreen as you inhale. Exhale . . . reach for your toes; breathe normally, applying sunscreen and gently massaging it on your toes, feet, legs, belly, back, shoulders, arms and hands, face, and ears.

PUT ON SUNGLASSES: Make a circle by touching the tip of your index finger and your thumb and place it over your eyes. You look fabulous! Now try on different-sized glasses, tapping each fingertip to the thumb tip until you find the ones that fit you best.

SET UP BEACH UMBRELLA: Standing Crescent Pose (page 44)

OPEN BEACH UMBRELLA: Tree (page 73)

Warm-Up

EXPLORE THE BEACH: Basic Sun Salutation (page 153). Guide your child to move through three rounds of Sun Salutations, using the following beach theme.

- **STAND ON BEACH:** Mountain (page 42). Feel the sand under your feet, breathe, and enjoy the fresh ocean air.

- **REACH FOR THE SUN:** Extended Mountain (page 43)

- **PLAY IN THE SAND:** Standing Forward Fold (page 46)

- **TEST THE WATER:** Low Lunge (page 53)—right side. Step one toe in and test the water!

- **STEP THE OTHER FOOT IN:** Plank (page 88)

- **GET YOUR WHOLE BODY WET:** Modified Low Push-Up (page 89)

- BODY SURF: Cobra (page 92). Here comes a wave, lift up your head and ride that wave!

- BIG WAVE: Downward Facing Dog (page 96). Whoa, here comes a huge wave!

- WASH ASHORE: Low Lunge—left side.

- BACK TO THE SAND: Standing Forward Fold. Step back on dry land; feel the sand!

- REACH FOR THE SUN: Extended Mountain. The sun will help you dry off.

- ENJOY THE MOMENT: Mountain. Take a breath and relax.

Wow, that was fun; let's go again! Repeat Basic Sun Salutation at least two more times to warm up!

Yoga Adventure

GO SURFING

- PADDLE OUT: Modified Locust with bilateral movement (page 105). Paddle out to catch a wave.

- BALANCE ON SURFBOARD: Warrior II (page 55)—right side!

- CATCH A WAVE: Reverse Warrior (page 56). Ride the wave all the way in to shore!

- Repeat "Go surfing" on the left side.

SNORKEL ADVENTURE

- SNORKEL BREATH: Breathe in, place snorkel (straw) in your mouth, and breathe out through the straw. What do you see on your snorkel trip?

TIP: Cue snorkel breath as a transition between each of the following poses:

- **Swimming starfish:** Triangle (page 57)
- **Cone-spiral shell:** Eagle (page 71)
- **Dolphin:** Dolphin (page 98)
- **Coiled shell:** Child's Pose (page 111)
- **Fish:** Locust (half, page 104). Lift only the upper body and swish your hands like fins; make a fish face.
- **Shark:** Locust (page 104)
- **Seahorse:** Rabbit (page 110). Tuck your toes to create a curly tail.
- **Crab:** Reverse Table (page 82). Walk sideways like a crab!
- **Octopus:** Standing or Seated Wide Leg Twist (page 60)
- **Clamshell:** Wide Leg Forward Fold (page 59)
- **Swimming Whale:** Whale Breath (page 130)
- **Gliding Whale:** Double Knee Reclined Twist (page 130)

RETURN TO BEACH

- REST ON TOWEL: Final Resting Pose (page 132)
- BUILD A SAND CASTLE: Roll back and forth between Plow (page 124) and Seated Forward Fold (page 32) poses.
- MAKE SAND ANGELS: Final Resting Pose—open arms and legs in star shape on inhale, draw legs together and arms alongside torso on exhale—move back and forth, creating sand angels.

Relaxation

Relax and dry off in sun. Take a big rest following all of that surfing, swimming, snorkeling, and playing.

PARTNER YOGA
Tweens (9–12 years)

Partner yoga is a lot of fun and sends a strong message to tweens to support each other, interact with each other, communicate clearly, see each other, and be there for each other. Parents can practice partner yoga with their child by simply making adjustments, where needed, and using props such as straps to compensate for differences in body size.

Music

Music with a positive message, gentle pop or lounge, instrumental, or jazz covers of popular songs are great for tween and teen yoga. Instrumental piano and nature sounds are also quite popular. Give your child a choice when it comes to her music (and yoga practice), for example, "What would you like to listen to? I have 'nature sounds,' 'gentle piano,' or 'mellow pop.'" By offering a choice of pre-edited playlists, the music will remain suitable for yoga, and your child will feel a sense of control and ownership of her yoga session.

Centering and Connecting with Your Partner

SEE *EACH OTHER*

- **SEE YOUR PARTNER:** Easy Pose (page 26). Greet your partner with a smile!
- **CONNECT WITH EACH OTHER:** Sunshine Breath (page 139). Practice three rounds of Sunshine Breath, connecting with your own breath; now practice three rounds of Sunshine Breath, syncing movement and breath with your partner.

Yoga Adventure

COMMUNICATE *AND* INTERACT *WITH EACH OTHER*

- **TWIN CRESCENT MOON:** Standing Crescent Pose (page 44). Stand side by side in Mountain (page 42). Move through three full rounds of Standing Crescent Pose, syncing movements and breath with your partner.

- FULL MOON: Remain standing side by side and release the arm closest to your partner so it rests alongside your torso. Circle outer arm around and overhead, linking hands with your partner to make a full moon.

- WAXING AND WANING MOON: Maintain gripped hands overhead and hold your partner's other hand. Inhale to prepare; as both of you exhale, rotate your bodies away from each other and circle arms to switch positions. You will both end up facing the other direction—the arms that were originally overhead now rest alongside your torso, and vice versa. Keep moving this way, waxing and waning for three full moon cycles.

- CHAIR LIFTS: Face your partner and grip each other's wrists. Inhale to straighten your arms fully and lean away from each other. Exhale: Lower into Chair Pose (page 68); hold and breathe in Chair Pose or practice Chair lifts—straightening the legs to rise on each inhale, lowering into Chair Pose on each exhale.

- TWISTING CHAIR: Face your partner and inhale, reaching your right arm straight up. Exhale and reach your right hand toward your partner's right hand, and grip each other's wrists. Inhale to lean away from each other and exhale. Continue leaning away from your partner as you bend your knees into Chair Pose. Open your left arm behind you, twisting your torso to the left. Inhale to rise, straightening your legs and reaching your left arm straight up overhead. As you exhale, switch your grip to the left wrist and lower into Chair Pose, reaching your right arm far behind you and opening your torso toward the right. Move back and forth, syncing your movement and breath with your partner's and supporting each other.

- SPAGHETTI-ARMED WARRIORS: Set up right-side Warrior I (page 50). Facing your partner, align your front (right) thigh so it is parallel to your partner's. Reach arms overhead and hold Warrior I. Extend your right hand toward your partner's right hip: Bend your left elbow, looping it behind your back to grip your partner's right wrist with your left hand (straps can be helpful if hands don't connect). Inhale to lengthen your upper body and gently lean away from each other on the exhale—only move the upper body and maintain strong Warrior I legs as you lean your torso away from your partner. Repeat on the left side.

- **WARRIOR TWINS:** Set up right-side Warrior II (page 55), so you are back to back with your partner (one partner will have the right leg forward and the other will have the left leg forward).

- **TWIN SURFERS:** Reverse Warrior (page 56)

- **TRIANGLE TWINS:** Straighten your forward-facing leg and move with your partner into Triangle (page 57).

- **REPEAT WARRIOR II–REVERSE WARRIOR–TRIANGLE**—left side! Switching directions with your partner is easy—maintain back-to-back alignment and reposition your feet so your back foot becomes the forward-facing foot, and vice versa.

- **LEANING PYRAMID:** Wide Leg Forward Fold (page 59). Begin in a wide-leg stance, back to back with your partner and a space of 1 to 2 feet between you. Inhale; reach your arms to shoulder height. Exhale; fold into Wide Leg Forward Fold. Reach your hands through your legs to grip your partner's wrists. Pull on each other's arms to lengthen your torsos away from each other and deepen the stretch.

SUPPORT *EACH OTHER*:

- **DOUBLE DOG:** Partner one begins in Downward Facing Dog (page 96). Partner two stands in front of partner one, facing forward. Partner two moves into Standing Forward Fold (page 46) and places both palms firmly on the floor; lifting one foot at a time, he gently places them onto partner one's sacrum (lower back) area, creating a Down Dog shape, with his feet on his partner's lower back and his hands on the floor in front of his partner. Hold for a few rounds of breath and switch.

- FLYING WARRIOR: Face your partner and grip each other's wrists. Step back until your arms are fully extended. Tip forward, lifting one leg off the ground to create Warrior III (page 62). Support each other in flying warrior for a few rounds of breath before switching legs.

- TWIN TREE: Stand side by side in Mountain Pose. Reach the inner arms straight up overhead and press your palms together. Bend the elbow of your outer arm and reach your forearm and hand across your chest to connect palm to palm with your partner in the middle. Stand strong on the inner leg (the one closest to your partner), and prop the outer leg into Tree Pose (page 73, foot resting at the ankle, calf, or inner thigh). Support each other in Tree Pose for a few rounds of breath. Face the other direction or switch sides with your partner to repeat on the other leg.

- DANCING DUET: Face your partner and create King of the Dancers Pose (page 76). Connect the palm of the raised arm with your partner's and press into each other's palms for support. Switch sides.

BE *THERE FOR EACH OTHER:*

- CAVE CRAWL: Partner one creates and holds Upward Facing Bow (page 117), while partner two crawls on his belly to pass underneath. Switch roles.

- DOUBLE-HUMPED CAMEL: Standing on your knees, face your partner. Both partners move into Camel (page 108), creating the two humps of a camel.

- SEESAW: Sit on the floor facing your partner in Staff Pose (page 30), with feet touching, if possible (if one partner has long legs, he can straddle his partner's legs). Reach forward and link hands around each other's wrists. Partner one gently leans back and pulls partner two into a Seated Forward Fold (page 32); partner two then leans back and gently pulls partner one into a Seated Forward Fold. Move back and forth with your partner, linking movement to breath: Inhale to rise and exhale to lean back/forward in either direction.

- TWIN-ENGINE BOAT: Sit facing your partner with toes touching, feet flat on floor, and knees bent. Reach your hands outside of your legs and link wrists with your partner. Press the soles of your feet into your partner's, and lift one leg at a time, until you are both in Boat Pose (page 34) with your feet connected to your partner's.

- SPAGHETTI NOODLE TWIST: Sit in Easy Pose (page 26), facing your partner so that your knees touch. Reach your right hand to the outside of your partner's right hip. Bend your left elbow and loop your forearm behind your back, connecting your left hand with your partner's right wrist (straps are an option). Inhale to lengthen your spine and sit up tall. Maintain that length as you exhale and lean away from your partner to twist to the left. Return to Easy Pose, switch, and repeat on the other side.

- FLIPPED TURTLE: Partner one becomes the turtle shell by creating Child's Pose (page 111). Partner two crouches near partner one's feet, facing away, and gently leans back, connecting his back with partner one's back. If partner one is comfortable, partner two can stretch out his arms and legs, resting his body on partner one—he is the soft part of the turtle stretching out. Switch roles.

- TWIN FALLS: Both partners create Waterfall (page 122), with legs straight up in the air and resting against their partner's legs. This requires a little communication and works best when one partner assumes the pose first, and then the second partner assumes the pose as if he were doing the same pose against the wall, coming as close to his partner's Waterfall as possible, and swinging his legs up to meet his partner's. Partner two may need to shuffle on his butt to get close enough to rest his legs against his partner's.

Relaxation

- BELLY PILLOWS: Partner one lies on his back; partner two rests his head on partner one's belly, resting on his back, perpendicular to partner one. Partner one practices Belly Breathing (page 140) with the weight of partner two's head adding resistance. Switch roles after about 5 minutes.

RESTORATIVE YOGA
Teens and Young Adults (13–18 years)

The following class plan includes a gentle to moderate warm-up sequence to get your teen or young adult up and moving. It is balanced with a number of restorative postures (a passive style of yoga combining use of props, body positioning, and gravity to stretch the body) to effectively stretch and support tight teens who are experiencing rapid growth spurts and bodily changes.

Suggested Props

- Bolsters (cushions or pillows)
- Blankets (large beach or bath towels)
- Straps (belts)
- Eye pillow

Music

See suggestions for Partner Yoga (page 206).

Centering

- Soothing Breath (page 137)

Warm-Up

- ROCK 'N' ROLL (page 119): Massage and stimulate the spine, back, and core muscles, rocking and rolling at least five times.
- EASY POSE (page 26): Find stillness.
- HIP CIRCLES (page 151): Move slowly and intentionally five times in each direction.
- TABLE (page 81): Align and lengthen your spine.

- CAT-COW FLOW (page 152): Warm up with five full rounds of Cat-Cow Flow.
- CHILD'S POSE-DOG FLOW (page 152): Continue warming up with Child-Dog Flow for five full rounds.
- BASIC SUN SALUTATION (page 153): Continue warm-up and meditation by flowing through five full rounds of Basic Sun Salutation.

TIP: Cue slow flow for Sun Salutation, allowing teens to take several breaths to move through each transition of Sun Salutation. Transition to Easy Pose (page 26).

Restore and Relax Yoga Stretches

Hold each pose for a minimum of five full rounds of breath to encourage deep relaxation.

- SEATED LATERAL BEND (page 45): Hold on each side or flow between sides, linking movement to breath.
- Transition to Staff Pose (page 30).
- SUPPORTED SEATED FORWARD FOLD (page 33)
- WIDE LEG FORWARD FOLD MODIFICATION (page 59)
- Transition to Table Pose (page 81).
- THREAD THE NEEDLE (page 86)
- Transition to prone position.
- CROCODILE (page 103)
- SUPPORTED CHILD'S POSE (page 113)
- Transition to Downward Facing Dog (page 96).
- HALF PIGEON (page 100)

Tip: If your teen is super tight, cue Reclined Pigeon variation (page 101).

- Transition to supine position.
- RECLINED BOUND ANGLE (page 29): Deep Belly Breathing (page 140) will help you relax in this pose.

- SUPPORTED BRIDGE (page 116)

- WATERFALL (page 122): Move directly from Supported Bridge into Waterfall. Simply straighten the legs and raise the feet toward the ceiling; sacrum rests on your support, and toes flex toward the face. You have the option to move to a wall and practice Legs Up the Wall variation (page 123).

- SUPPORTED FISH (page 129): Place bolster beneath shoulder blades; if neck is hyperextended, use a pillow to support the head and reduce hyperextension of the neck.

- KNEES TO CHEST (page 118)

- HAPPY BABY (page 120)

- WIND RELIEVING POSE (page 121)

- DOUBLE KNEE RECLINED TWIST (page 130)

- FINAL RESTING POSE (page 132): Be sure your teen is super supported with pillows, blankets, and an eye pillow. Dim the lights and play relaxing music to help your teen rest and restore.

CHAPTER SEVEN

Connect:
Yoga Games

So much more than fun and play, yoga games are a creative way for kids to explore, review, and lead yoga poses. They are also beneficial to a child's physical, sensory, cognitive, and social development. In Sanskrit, the word *yoga* means "to yoke or connect." The games in this chapter create a sense of community and support your child's connection with siblings, friends, and classmates.

This chapter features twenty-five yoga games, with a brief description of the benefits, supplies, and minimum number of players needed, along with instructions on how to play. You may recognize childhood favorites and discover traditional games that have been reimagined to relate to yoga, I hope these inspire you and your child to invent your own yoga games. Parents can play games requiring a minimum of two players along with their child, and if you have a large group, of course you can explore all the games as a whole or by splitting up players into smaller groups.

Benefits of Yoga Games

» **BILATERAL COORDINATION:** Intentional movement of both sides of the body in unison, for example, raising the right arm and lifting the left leg at the same time

» **GROSS MOTOR PLANNING:** Function of the brain to understand, plan, and organize a logical sequence of actions that incorporate large body parts—arms, legs, torso, and head—to carry out a task

» **MENTAL FUNCTION:** Ability to think, plan, understand, reason, perceive, imagine, and recall

» **SENSORY INPUT:** Stimuli perceived by the sensory system. In the case of vestibular, tactile, and proprioceptive input indicates body position (sitting, lying, standing), movement (speed, direction, etc.), and balance.

» **SENSORY PROCESSING:** Ability of the brain to interpret sensory input and organize an appropriate response

» **PROPRIOCEPTIVE:** Sense that pertains to body position and movement

» **VESTIBULAR:** Sense that pertains to balance and movement

» **TACTILE:** Sense that pertains to touch

NAME THAT BEANBAG

BENEFITS: Focus, concentration, present moment awareness, mental function, coordination, hand-eye coordination

You will need

- Small beanbags in a variety of shapes and colors

💬 Simple Steps for Kids

- Select a beanbag and stand facing your partner (be sure you each have a beanbag of a different color or shape).
- Toss your beanbag to your partner and call its color or shape as you do.
- Your partner will do the same.
- Increase the challenge—call out the color or shape of the beanbag you are catching as well as the one you are throwing!
- Increase the challenge even more—toss your beanbag at the same time as your partner!

TIP: This game can get loud, but it's a lot of fun, and kids are 100 percent in the moment while playing.

WHEELBARROW GAME

BENEFITS: Bilateral coordination, motor planning, weight bearing, upper body and core strengthening, teamwork, communication, cooperation

Tips for Parents/Teachers

- Create a wheelbarrow course by lining up yoga mats. Place items for your child to collect along the way—flash cards or something that kids can easily place in a pocket and bring back to the beginning of the course.

- After playing wheelbarrow, create yoga poses based on the items collected.

 ## Simple Steps for Kids

- Partner with a friend who is similar in height and decide who will start as the wheelbarrow and who will be the driver. Remember, you will switch and play both roles!

- The wheelbarrow positions himself on all fours, and the driver stands behind him, facing forward.

- The wheelbarrow lifts and straightens one leg at a time, and the driver takes a grip of each lower calf, just above the ankles, to support the wheelbarrow.

- Work together to move around the room, or follow a course if one has been set! Wheelbarrows walk on the palms, and drivers walk behind.

- Switch roles.

- Once everybody has had a turn being the wheelbarrow, work with a partner or in small groups to create yoga poses based on the cards or items you collected along the way. Take turns leading the yoga poses with your peers.

BASKET-BEANBAG

BENEFITS: Focus, centering, hand-eye coordination

You will need

- Small beanbags
- Images of basketball hoops marked with numbers 1, 2, and 3
- Tape

 Simple Steps for Kids

- Tape images of basketball hoops (photo or flash-card size) at one end of a yoga mat. Be sure to stagger them according to point value: 1 point is a free shot—place it front and center. Place the images of the second two hoops a little farther away. If you like, angle them slightly to increase the challenge. The image of the hoop with a value of 3 points should be the most challenging.
- Stand at the opposite end of the yoga mat.
- Begin with three beanbags and toss them toward the markers. Tally your score.
- Practice for a few rounds and see how well you do on your own before learning the "yoga trick."

Yoga Trick for Kids!

Relax and center your mind and body before you play! Try this: Inhale as you take aim and prepare to toss your beanbag. . . . Exhale as you mindfully toss your beanbag toward the markers. Did this help improve your score?

BUTTERFLY ROLL*/HOT DOG/BURRITO ROLL

BENEFITS: Vestibular, tactile input, core strengthening

You will need

- One yoga mat

 Simple Steps for Kids

- Place a yoga mat horizontally on the floor, preferably on a soft, padded surface (such as a carpet or rug) in an open space.
- Lie on your back at one end of the mat, aligning your shoulders with the horizontal (long) edge. This step is important so that your head and face remain exposed once you are rolled up in the mat.
- Zip your legs together and press your arms against your torso, like a tin solider.
- Ask a parent or friend to gently roll your body, bundling you in the yoga mat.
- You're a caterpillar in his cocoon. Imagine what colors your wings will be when you become a butterfly.
- When you feel ready to become a butterfly, make yourself as stiff as a tin soldier. Ask your parent or friend to hold the short end of the yoga mat and gently pull on it, rolling you—the beautiful butterfly—out of his cocoon.

TIP: If your child does not wish to be a butterfly, he could be a hot dog or burrito! Check in with your child as you are rolling him in the mat, as he may be claustrophobic. In that case, you can roll him very loosely in the mat and be ready to unroll him immediately if he begins to indicate that he is not comfortable.

MEMORY GAME

BENEFITS: Introduces the concept of intuition, supports memory, focus, patience

You will need

- Flash cards with duplicate images (pairs)

 Simple Steps for Kids

- Shuffle the cards well and place them facedown on the floor.
- Elect a starter. This person flips any two cards, and, if a match is revealed, he keeps the cards and takes another turn.
- If a match is not revealed, he flips the cards back over, and the next person will go.
- At the end of the game, take turns creating and leading yoga poses based on the images from your collected cards.

MUSICAL MATS

BENEFITS: Communication, listening skills, cooperation

You will need

- Cards with names or images of yoga poses
- One yoga mat per card (or one yoga mat per child)
- Tape

 Simple Steps for Kids

- Set mats around the room—they do not need to be perfectly arranged and can be placed in different angles and positions.
- Tape a yoga pose card to the floor at the top of each mat.
- Ask a parent or teacher to be in charge of music. When the music plays, dance around the room.
- When the music stops, find the closest yoga mat and create the pose on the card at the top of the mat.

or

- Set up enough mats so everybody has one.
- When the music stops, find a yoga mat and strike a yoga pose of your choice (no cards or tape required!).

TIP: Be sure to allow enough time for children to find their expression of each pose and hold it before restarting the music.

FOOTBALL

BENEFITS: Core strength, coordination, motor planning

You will need

- A small- to medium-size ball (or small beanbag)

 Simple Steps for Kids

- Pass the ball back and forth with a partner or around a circle in a group, using only the feet!

TOE-GA

BENEFITS: Stretches the toes and feet, core strengthening, coordination, motor planning

You will need

- Pom-poms of varying sizes (or cotton balls)

 Simple Steps for Kids

- Pick up a pom-pom using your toes and pass it back and forth with a partner or around a group circle.
- Remember you can only use your toes!

AIR-MAZING

BENEFITS: Core strengthening, proprioceptive and tactile input, lip positioning/closure (to support speech development), breath control

You will need

- Yoga bolsters and blocks, or something similar, for the maze
- Pom-poms or cotton balls
- Drinking straws

 Simple Steps for Kids

- Set up a maze using props to build barriers and dead ends, or ask a friend or teacher to set one up for you so you can solve it!
- Lie on your belly at the starting point and, blowing through a straw, move a pom-pom through the entire maze, using only your breath.

TIP: Gauge a safe distance between children following each other through the maze.

YOGI SAYS

BENEFITS: Listening, communication and leadership skills, review of yoga poses

You will need

- Cards with yoga pose images (optional, for kids who may be stuck for inspiration)

 Simple Steps for Kids

- Elect a leader.
- The leader guides her peers to create a yoga pose of her choosing.
- As with the game Simon Says, if she uses the phrase, "Yogi says," the group follows her instruction. If the leader offers a cue without saying "Yogi says" and somebody follows her, the leader gets a point!
- Continue until the yoga pose is complete and switch leaders. Whoever has the most points at the end of the game is the queen/king of Yogi Says!

TIP: The leader gains a point if a mistake is made—this way nobody is "out" and each yoga pose can be fully experienced.

ANIMAL, VEGETABLE, MINERAL

BENEFITS: Mental processing, identification and organization skills, communication skills

In this game, an elected leader creates a yoga pose and the class must guess what it is and categorize it as animal, vegetable, or mineral.

 ## Simple Steps for Kids

- Elect a leader. The leader must create a yoga pose based on an animal, mineral, or vegetable.

- The class must identify what the yoga pose represents, and which category it falls under. For example, if the leader is demonstrating Bound Angle Pose (page 27), and you decide she is a butterfly, it would fall in the animal category.

- The member of the group who identifies the object and places it into the correct category is the winner and leads the next pose.

- For extra fun, create a pose for each category and provide the correct answer using yoga—for example, Lion's Breath animal, Tree vegetable, and Child's Pose mineral (rock).

EGG 'N' SPOON

BENEFITS: Coordination, balance, focus, mindful movement

You will need

- Spoons
- Plastic eggs or hard-boiled eggs
- Obstacle course made with tape, yoga mats, or traffic cones

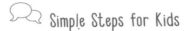 Simple Steps for Kids

- Carefully balance an egg on your spoon and carefully walk along the course.
- If you drop your egg, you must go back to the start!
- Check your breath! Are you breathing or holding your breath? Even the most challenging game is easier when you breathe!

TIP: Turn this game into a yoga class—use plastic eggs with toys inside! After finishing the course, the kids can open their eggs to reveal the toys. Lead a prepared sequence (i.e., parents, be sure to plan a yoga sequence based on the toys inside the eggs *before* playing this game), or ask kids to create their own yoga poses for the toys inside their eggs.

YOGA TWISTER

BENEFITS: Memory recall, balance, coordination, creativity, flexibility, review of yoga poses

 ## Simple Steps for Kids

- Elect a leader.

- The leader calls out different body parts at random.

- Peers create a yoga pose with only those body parts touching the floor.

- For example, if the leader calls "butt," you could create Boat Pose; if the leader calls "one foot," you could create Tree, Dancer, Warrior III, or any pose that requires you to balance on one foot!

The following games work best with a minimum of three players and can easily be adapted for larger groups.

HOT YOGA POTATO

BENEFITS: Listening, communication and leadership skills, patience

You will need

- Single beanbag or similar item
- Music—the adult should have access to the source in order to pause it at random intervals (as you would if you were playing Musical Chairs)

Simple Steps for Kids

- Sit in a circle with your friends and pass a beanbag from one person to the next. Don't hold it—it's a hot potato!
- Ask a parent or teacher to play music, pausing it randomly.
- When the music stops, whoever is holding the hot potato leads the group through a yoga pose of her choosing.
- Once the pose is complete (on both sides, to be balanced), take your seats and recommence the game beginning with the child seated next to the leader.

TIP: For core strengthening, use the feet instead of the hands to pass the beanbag!

DOWN-DOG TUNNEL

BENEFITS: Teamwork, communication, coordination, gross-motor planning, proprioceptive and tactile input, upper body and core strengthening

 ## Simple Steps for Kids

- Line up, side by side, on all fours, facing the same direction and close enough to almost touch your neighbor on each side.

- On the count of three, create Downward Facing Dog (page 96) together, making a Downward Facing Dog tunnel.

- The child at the end steps out of the pose and crawls through the tunnel on his belly. When he reaches the end of the tunnel, he rejoins it by assuming Downward Facing Dog Pose.

- Take turns moving down the tunnel, one child at a time, until everybody has had a turn.

- If somebody gets tired, she must say, "Doggy rest!" Everybody takes a rest in Table (page 81) or Child's Pose (page 111). Obviously, this cannot occur while a friend is crawling through the tunnel; wait until she has passed under your section of the tunnel. Or, if you notice you are beginning to feel tired, give her the heads-up and call "Doggy rest" before she begins to crawl through the tunnel.

TIP: This game can be altered to suit the theme of your yoga class, for example, make a dinosaur cave for dinosaur yoga. Encourage children to communicate with one another if they begin to run out of space. They will need to shuffle their bodies along to keep the tunnel in the same place.

BELL GAME

BENEFITS: Focus, concentration, cooperation, patience, mindfulness

You will need

- **Small bell on a string or ribbon**

 Simple Steps for Kids

- Sit in a circle.
- Place the bell on the floor in front of the person who will start the game.
- The person with the bell in front of him must pick it up and stand without the bell ringing. He will then carefully walk and place the bell on the floor in front of another friend in the circle—without ringing the bell!
- Once the bell has been placed, the player returns to his place in the circle and sits quietly listening for the bell as the next person tries to move it without making a sound.

ISLAND GAME

BENEFITS: Communication, teamwork, listening skills, cooperation

You will need

- One yoga mat per child

 Simple Steps for Kids

- Scatter yoga mats around the room.

- Ask a parent or teacher to play music, stopping it randomly.

- Dance around the room—when the music stops, find a yoga mat and create a yoga pose on the mat.

- Ask your parent or teacher to take one yoga mat out of the game after each round. When the music stops, you will need to begin *sharing* mats, working together to create poses that allow you to fit on one mat together.

- Eventually, there will be just one mat remaining and you will need to work together to find a pose that allows you all to share the mat (hint: Mountain Pose works well for large groups).

ROLLER-COASTER RIDE

BENEFITS: Core strength, coordination, teamwork, cooperation, communication

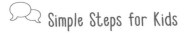 Simple Steps for Kids

- Sit single file in a row, facing forward, straddling the person in front of you with your legs.
- Reach your arms forward to link with the person in front of you.
- The person at the back of the row "steers" the roller coaster.
- To climb the peak, lean back—gently pulling back the person in front of you.
- Lean forward to go down the roller coaster and lean to either side to take corners.
- Have fun! Raise your arms in air and ask your friends to do the same—see how long your core strength, teamwork, and communication can maintain this wild and crazy roller-coaster ride!

TIP: This game works best for small groups of four to six, but it can be a lot of fun and generate plenty of laughs with larger groups.

YOGA CHARADES

BENEFITS: Teamwork, verbal and nonverbal communication, leadership skills, recall/memory, review of yoga poses, steps to create yoga poses

You will need

- Images of yoga poses (optional, for kids who may feel stuck when called upon)

 Simple Steps for Kids

- Select a leader.
- The leader directs peers, step by step, through a yoga pose of her choosing without talking!
- Follow the leader step by step. Can you guess what yoga pose she is demonstrating?
- The person who guesses the pose before it is complete earns a point and will lead the next round. The leader completes leading the pose before switching leaders.
- If nobody guesses the name of the pose, or it is not identified until the pose is complete, the leader earns a point and remains leader of the next round.
- The person with the most points at the end of the game is the yoga charade champion!

HUMAN MANDALA

BENEFITS: Teamwork, communication, connection, creativity

Mandala is Sanskrit for *circle*. Mandalas are a simple or intricate design contained within a circle. Usually quite colorful, they are used as a focal point for meditation. Human mandalas are a fun way for kids to connect with one another and work as a team to create beautiful mandala designs using their bodies.

You will need

- Groups of three or more work best for this game, but it is a lot of fun in larger groups, too!

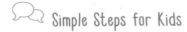

Simple Steps for Kids

- Work together to create simple or complex shapes in a circle using your body.
- Be sure the pattern repeats itself and the circle is complete and symmetrical in design . . . just like a mandala!

Here are some suggestions to get you started:

- CANDY CANE MANDALA: Lie side by side, forming a circle, with your feet touching at the center. Reach your arms overhead and curl to the left, like a candy cane. Switch directions and curl to the right.

- LOTUS FLOWER MANDALA: Sit in a circle in Bound Angle Pose (page 27), knees connecting with your neighbor on either side. Turn your palms to face out and connect palm to palm with the person on each side of you. Inhale, reach your hands up, pressing into each other's palms; exhale to lower hands back down. Move together, synchronizing your breath to create a lotus flower opening and closing.

- **SLEEPING BUTTERFLY MANDALA:** Begin sitting in a circle in Bound Angle Pose. Lie on your back in Reclined Bound Angle (page 29). Reach your arms out and link them with the person on each side of you. Relax.
- **DANCING MANDALA:** Sit in a circle in Staff Pose (page 30), feet meeting in the middle. Reach arms overhead and breathe in, exhale into a Seated Forward Fold (page 32). Inhale back through Staff Pose, with arms raised overhead, and exhale lowering arms as you roll back into Plow Pose (page 124). Move back and forth from Plow to Staff to Seated Forward Fold and back again, syncing your breath and movements with your friends.

HULA HOOP LINK

BENEFITS: Teamwork, communication, cooperation, motor planning, coordination

You will need

- One hula hoop per group of children

 Simple Steps for Kids

- Form a circle, holding hands with the person on each side of you.
- One person releases a hand to loop a hula hoop onto his arm, reconnecting hands to close the circle.
- Work as a team passing the hula hoop around the circle without breaking the link. Communicate with one another and use your arms, shoulders, heads, and legs to pass your body through the hoop, moving it to the person next to you.
- Switch directions.

BIRD ON A STRING

BENEFITS: Teamwork, communication, connection, creativity, breath control, balance

You will need

- Large button
- Colorful feathers
- Glue
- Twine
- Three players per group

Simple Steps for Kids

- **MAKE YOUR BIRD:** Glue two feathers on a large button to make your "button- bird." Allow the glue to set before playing.

- **BIRD ON A STRING:** Players one and two become trees, standing a few yards from each other, holding a piece of twine taut between them. (Challenge yourself! Hold Tree Pose, page 73, if you are player one or two.)

- Thread the first button-bird on the length of twine, close to one of the "trees."

- Player three becomes the wind. The wind must help the button-bird to fly by gently and steadily blowing it from one tree to the other.

- Once the wind blows the bird all the way to the second tree, remove the bird from the string and replace it with the next player's bird.

- Switch until each player has played the wind, and each tree has caught a bird.

- Try different breathing techniques to see which helps your bird fly better. Does a short, sharp burst of breath move your bird? Or is a nice long, steady breath better?

- Notice, too, how you feel acting as the wind! If the wind gets tired, the bird will never make it across—find a breath that moves the bird without tiring you out! If the bird's feathers get ruffled, it may get mad. We don't want that, so find a breath that works for the bird and the wind . . . and the poor old trees holding Tree Pose!

LAST YOGI STANDING

BENEFITS: Stamina, flexibility, strength, confidence, mindfulness

 Simple Steps for Kids

- Choose a yoga pose that is challenging to hold (balance poses are great for this game).
- Hold the pose for as long as you can.
- The last person holding the pose will be crowned as "last yogi standing" and chooses the next pose to challenge the group.

TIP: Vary poses according to your child's ability. Be sure to offer poses on both sides for balance!

The following games require four or more players, and can be adapted for even larger groups.

HIDE THE BEANBAG

BENEFITS: Introduces the concept of intuition, awareness of body language, nonverbal cues

You will need

- One small beanbag per group
- Small groups of four or five children work best for this game.

Simple Steps for Kids

- Begin sitting in a circle with your friends and one small beanbag.

- Select one person from your group to step away, out of sight and hearing range.

- While this person is away, elect another member of your group to hide the beanbag. It must remain in the group, hidden, so that it is not visible. For example, place it in a pocket or sit on it.

- Call the friend, who stepped away, back to your circle. He must use his intuition to figure out who has the beanbag. He can take as many "intuitive" guesses as he needs. Once he correctly identifies the child with the beanbag, he and the child trade places. Continue playing until everybody has stepped away and used their intuitive skills to locate the beanbag.

WEB OF LOVE

BENEFITS: Awareness of self and of peers, compassion, empathy, unity, self-esteem, self-confidence

You will need

- Ball of wool or twine
- One wooden craft stick per child (optional)
- Small groups of five or six children work best for this game, allowing each child to receive several compliments.

 Simple Steps for Kids

- Begin sitting in a circle and elect a "starter" person to hold the ball of wool.
- The starter wraps the end piece of wool loosely around his hand and holds onto it. He then rolls the ball of wool to another participant, along with a verbal compliment—for example, "Cindy, you are amazing at basketball."
- The participant receiving the compliment loosely loops a section of twine around her hand before rolling ball to another participant, along with a verbal compliment, "John, you have a great smile."
- Continue until a giant web appears.

TIP: Give each child a craft stick to wrap the twine around each time they receive a compliment. The web can then be transferred to a wall as a creative and artful reminder of how wonderful each individual child is, and how connected they are as a group. Decorate the web with sticky notes highlighting the compliments each child received from his peers.

Acknowledgments

This book would be nothing more than thoughts, lesson plans, and teaching experience stored in my memory bank if not for Meredith Hale, who encouraged me to shape my ideas into words on paper; and the talented team at Sterling who took those pages and turned them into the beautifully finished book that you hold in your hands today.

A special thank you to my editor at Sterling, Jennifer Williams, your insight, kindness, and encouragement throughout each stage of production has been unwavering, and greatly appreciated.

The fun illustrations and gorgeous design are credited to creative team, Julia Morris, Shannon Plunkett, and Elizabeth Lindy, who demonstrated patience and grace working with a stickler for alignment in yoga poses (me!). Big thanks also go to production editor Renee Yewdaev for skillfully keeping everything on course.

And finally, the children I have had the honor to work with. I am so grateful for each one of you. Every day I am challenged to grow as a yoga teacher; my mind, imagination, and teaching skills are constantly evolving, because of and for you.

Index

Note: Page numbers in *italics* indicate poses or pose variations.

About the Author

Lisa Roberts is a registered yoga teacher and registered children's yoga teacher, and holds a certificate in children's yoga therapy. She has worked in the pediatric wellness field since 2006 and currently leads the in-patient yoga program at St. Louis Children's Hospital.

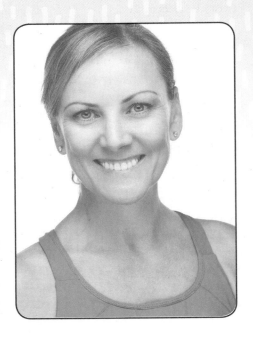

Lisa offers professional training, teaching Kids Adaptive and Accessible Yoga to pediatric professionals, parents, and yoga teachers. She is the author of *Teach Your Child Meditation* (Sterling 2018) and has developed a line of teaching tools for pediatric yoga teachers, parents, and kids, including a children's yoga storybook, guided breathing and relaxation CDs, and yoga flash cards.

WEBSITE: www.yoyoyogaschool.com
BLOG: http://yoyoyogaschool.com/teaching-tips/blog
FACEBOOK: https://www.facebook.com/yoyoyogaschool
TWITTER: @yoyoyogaschool